The Single Payer Healthcare System
- Faults and Fixes

Henry P. Krahn,
B. SC. (Med), M.D., F.R.C.S.(C).

◆ FriesenPress

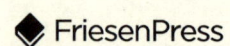

Suite 300 - 990 Fort St
Victoria, BC, Canada, V8V 3K2
www.friesenpress.com

Copyright © 2016 by Henry P. Krahn, B. SC. (Med), M.D., F.R.C.S.(C).
First Edition — 2016

All rights reserved.

No part of this publication may be reproduced in any form, or by any means, electronic or mechanical, including photocopying, recording, or any information browsing, storage, or retrieval system, without permission in writing from FriesenPress.

ISBN
978-1-4602-7888-8 (Hardcover)
978-1-4602-7889-5 (Paperback)
978-1-4602-7890-1 (eBook)

1. Medical, Medicaid & Medicare

Distributed to the trade by The Ingram Book Company

Quotation

"The best interest of the patient is the only interest to consider."
William J. Mayo

Author Dedication

THIS BOOK IS DEDICATED TO THE MEMORY OF THE LATE DR. JACK Hildes (1918-1984), Professor of Medicine at the University of Manitoba and founder of the Hildes Northern Medical Unit in Manitoba. Dr. Hildes was an inspiration, role model, mentor, and true friend of mine at a time when a medical career seemed to be just a distant, impossible dream.

Definitions

It is important to differentiate between Social Health Insurance and Socialized Medicine.

According to Uwe E. Rhinehart*, Social health Insurance refers to an insurance-based healthcare system. The providers submit bills to a government single-payer insurance carrier and get paid on a fee-for-service basis. Standard American Medicare is a good example of social health insurance.

Socialized medicine refers to a system in which the government not only pays for the healthcare programs but also manages them.

Canada started with social health insurance in the hospitals in 1958. In the 1970's, they switched to government-managed care in the hospital component of Medicare, or socialized medicine.

---

*   *Uwe E. Rhinehart, New York Times, May, 2009*

Table of Contents

Quotation	iii
Author Dedication	v
Definitions	vii
Introduction	1
Author's Professional Experience	7
Acknowledgments	11
Chapter 1: How Medicare Began in Canada	13
Chapter 2: Manitoba Health	21
Chapter 3: The Unit Cost of Service	31
Chapter 4: Scarcity and Rationing	33
Chapter 5: Wait List	47
Chapter 6: Quality Controls	55
Chapter 7: Lack of Incentives	67

Chapter 8:
Physician Issues   71

Chapter 9:
Personal Care Homes   95

Chapter 10:
The Prescription Pharmacy Plan   99

Chapter 11:
Controversial WRHA Decisions   101

Chapter 12:
Evidence-Based Medicine   105

Chapter 13:
Cook in another City   117

Chapter 14:
Canadian Life Expectancy   121

Chapter 15:
A Mandarin Snit   123

Chapter 16:
Horror Stories   125

Chapter 17:
Canadian Medicare Malaise   137

Chapter 18:
Seeking a Political Solution   141

Chapter 19:
Manitoba Health Mendacity   153

Chapter 20:
Building a Clinical Oligarchy   157

Chapter 21:
Over-regulation of Technology	163

Chapter 22:
National Insolvency with Medicare	167

Chapter 23:
Investigative Journalism	171

Chapter 24:
American Healthcare Systems	175

Chapter 25:
Reforming the American Healthcare System	185

Chapter 26:
Reforming the Canadian HealthCare System	199

Conclusion	221

Curriculum Vitae	223

List of Publications and Presentations	225

Book Published	233

About the Author	235

Introduction

One Day of Observing Canadian Medicare

ON AN EARLY JULY WEEKEND IN SUMMER, I WAS VISITED BY A COLleague from the US who trained with me in Bellevue Hospital, New York City. He was practicing about 300 miles south of Winnipeg. I offered to take him on my morning rounds at the hospital.

When we entered the hospital, near the ER, he wanted to know why there were three ambulances parked near the door. I approached the driver of the first ambulance and asked, "How long have you been here?" He replied, "close to three hours." "We have to wait until the ER accepts the patient." He continued, "Patients are triaged on the basis of medical need. If there are more urgent patients in the waiting room the ambulance crew has to wait. The patient is on the EMO gurney parked in the hallway with two attendants until he is officially handed over to the ER staff. Ours will be the next to be accepted, providing no one else shows up more urgent."

"Since there are so many ambulances tied up at the ER all the time, what happens when one is needed in an emergency?", my friend enquired. "That can be a problem," the EMO driver replied. "The Winnipeg Free Press reported an instance where a woman was injured in a crash on McPhillips Street and it took more than two hours for an ambulance to arrive." "There were 17 ambulances waiting to off-load patients at various ERs at the time."

The ER was crowded to the rafters, with people sitting on the floor and spilling out into the street. Some had waited for 10 or 11 hours to be seen. (Parenthetically, the Canadian Broadcasting Corporation (CBC) reported on September 14, 2014, one Winnipeg hospital had the worst wait times in the country – 90% waited more than 9 hours.)

I informed my friend from the US, "Ten per cent of patients leave without being seen. They get frustrated and disgusted and go home. Recently a woman left after waiting six hours and was found dead at home the next day from an epidural hematoma."

I continued, "There is so much mayhem in the ER that foolish decisions are sometimes made by the staff. In 2014, they sent two patients home from the ER by taxi at night, when the ambient temperature outside was 35 degrees below zero. One was sent home in his pajamas and bed-room slippers. They both froze to death on the street outside their homes."

My friend couldn't believe that. "Surely nobody in the ER would ever send anyone home without an escort in the middle of the night, or at least make sure there is somebody at home to receive them?" "Nope, evidently not," I replied.

When the Minister of Health was queried about this by the press, she maintained that no rules or protocols were breached. She reportedly said, "It was the fault of the taxi drivers – they should never leave a person on the street in his pajamas until they know the person is safe inside the house."

By now my American friend was shocked. "What about The Joint Commission on Hospital Accreditation (JCACHO)?" he asked. Every accredited hospital in the US has a JCACHO certificate posted prominently near the front entrance. JCACHO in the US inspects and certifies hospitals. They do regular annual inspections and also do unannounced inspections when there are complaints.

I responded, "In Canada there is no Joint Commission." "The government manages the hospital. The same government also inspects and sets standards. There is no third party level of regulation whatsoever." "When mistakes are made they are apt to be covered up."

Inside the ER it was bedlam. We did not go into the resuscitation area, but the corridors were lined with gurneys on both sides with a narrow passage in between. There were three ambulance crews lounging near their patients.

I asked one woman how long she had been there. She had fallen off a bicycle and had a comminuted fracture of her arm. They had told her on admission she would be operated on that day. At 8 pm she was told she would have to wait until tomorrow. The same thing happened the next day. This was her third day of waiting.

We spoke to another man who had been on a gurney in the ER for a whole week. He was going to be discharged that morning. He was there because of unstable heart problems. He spent a week in the ER with a life-threatening complaint and was never admitted to a hospital bed!

We went upstairs to the Urology ward to visit my patients.

He was shocked to see all the equipment stored in the hall. There was a portable electrocardiogram machine, a breathing machine with an Oxygen tank, an empty gurney, two patients on gurneys with intravenous tubes and various tables and chairs. My friend commented, "How does the Fire Marshal allow this?" "This is a fire hazard!"

When visiting a patient of mine recovering nicely from a radical cancer operation, he said he couldn't sleep last night. At 2 am they admitted a woman to the bed beside him (yes, opposite sexes share the same room), and she was so sick they rushed her to the operating room.

My urology colleague told me afterwards she had a stone obstructing her kidney. He tried to admit her all last week on an urgent basis because she had a urinary tract infection and low fever. He could not get her admitted. She suddenly became septicemic and he was just barely able to save her life that night. Endotoxic shock carries a mortality rate of 50%.

We passed a ward on the other side of the nurses station where there was nothing going on. The ward looked exactly like the urology ward except there were elderly patients in dressing gowns sitting in their lounges reading newspapers or watching television, as if they were at home. This was one of the many wards that harbored people waiting for a personal care home. Many of them had been there for almost two years. These are the boarders who occupy 39 per cent of all the acute care beds.

Lastly, I took him to another ward that was completely empty. This was July, the time of the six week closure. A third of the acute care beds are always closed during all of July and two weeks in August.

Afterward, I took my friend out to lunch at my club and we happened to sit with a gentleman who serves on the Board of the hospital. I asked him how much money is saved by closing all those beds during the summer. "Well, it's not that much," he replied. "We cannot lay off permanent staff. We keep people on temporary staff for as long as possible because those we can lay off. The maintenance of the building, the depreciation of equipment, and the servicing of debt don't take a holiday. I would estimate a six week closure saves us the cost of operating the hospital for a week, but certainly no more."

As we were walking back to our car, my friend seemed very quiet and deep in thought. I asked him, "What seems to be bothering you?"

He took a deep breath, paused a long time to collect himself, and finally made some sagacious observations. "I don't get it. Your ER reminds me of a hospital I worked in while in Africa, where I spent two years as a Peace Corps doctor. Patients used to start lining up at 4 am to be seen by the doctor at 10 am. Your hospital looks like it is flat broke. All those empty beds and those boarders are wasting precious resources. You have told me about the scarcity of beds and the horrendous wait lists. You must have thousands of people who cannot access expeditious, timely care. You likely have unnecessary suffering and doubtless many avoidable deaths. I look at the cars in the parking lot, the skyscrapers, the fancy restaurants and I don't get any sense of general poverty. There seems to be scarcity and hardship in healthcare in a land of plenty."

"You have hit the nail on the head," I said. "It's the system, my friend. It's called socialism." "85% of Canadians think this is wonderful, because it is free," I continued. "This is all that anyone under the age of 50 years has ever known. " "They feel good about it because they hear of medical bankruptcies in your country." They hear 40 million people in your country don't have access to healthcare." "But those are lies," my friend interjected. "Yes," I said, "You and I know they are lies, but that is what people over here are told and that is what they believe."

"I promise you one thing," I continued. "Someday I will write a book – an expose." "There is a better way." "When I retire I will write such a book." "Having lived and worked in both countries there is no one better positioned to write such a book."

Author's Professional Experience

HENRY P. KRAHN, M.D. GRADUATED FROM THE FACULTY OF Medicine, University of Manitoba in 1958. He interned at Winnipeg General Hospital (1958-1960), and then trained in urology at New York University-Bellevue Medical Centre (1960-1964). He was certified as a urology specialist in1964 in both Canada and the US.

After completing his training in New York City, Krahn looked forward to returning to Canada. He remembered the clean, well-run hospitals with an ample supply of modern facilities and bed capacity. There was a universal public hospital insurance plan in place, but the government did not manage the hospitals. The public had quick and trouble-free access to hospitals, and medical staff appointments were easy to obtain. The Canadian hospital system appeared superior to anything he had seen during his American medical residency.

Within a year of returning, Krahn was appointed Head of Urology at Children's Hospital in Winnipeg, which later became part of the Health Sciences Centre.

During that time he authored a landmark paper, "The Acute Scrotum", published in the prestigious *Journal of Urology*[*]. Torsion of the testicle typically occurs at puberty, when there is a sudden surge in the volume of the testicle. If the testicle is poorly attached

---

*   *Journal of Urology, 104: 601, 1970.*

to the sidewall of the scrotum (a variation of undescended testicle), the testicle can twist and the blood supply through the spermatic cord cut off. This kills the testicle in just a few hours. The congenital abnormality can be present on both sides. If both testicles are lost the boy would never develop male secondary sexual characteristics and will be infertile. In the mid1960s, there was limited imaging technology available, so the definitive diagnosis could only be made via surgical exploration. If too much time is spent dithering over the diagnosis, the testicle is usually lost.

There was a twenty-fold increase in the incidence of testicular torsion at Children's Hospital in Winnipeg during Krahn's tenure in Urology in the mid1960s. A retrospective review of the previous two years showed a similar number of boys sent home from the emergency department with a diagnosis of "inflamed testicle". The vast majority of these boys can be presumed to have suffered a testicular torsion, and subsequently lost at least one gonad.

The term "Acute Scrotum" coined by Krahn and co-author N.H. Moharib, M.D., stuck, and is still referenced in pediatric urology textbooks.

Soon after, Krahn was appointed Head of Urology at St. Boniface General Hospital (a 600-bed teaching hospital). Krahn served in that position for 23 years. Krahn's proudest achievement during his St. Boniface years was a paper he co-authored with M.V. Mathur, M.D. and E. W. Ramsey, M.D. on cancer of the bladder, also published in the *Journal of Urology*[*]. They reported their experience with radical surgery for bladder cancer with resultant low morbidity and no mortality. At that time urologists were engaged in a vigorous debate over the best treatment for bladder cancer. Most urologists favored radiotherapy for these cases. Krahn, and his associates, were among the first to report better success rates with radical surgery.

---

[*]   *Journal of Urology, June, 1981*

In recognition of these achievements, Krahn was appointed Associate Professor of Surgery (Urology) by the University of Manitoba. He was also Chief of Surgery at Concordia Hospital (a Winnipeg community hospital) for over 30 years. Krahn practiced urology in Manitoba for a total of 38 years. He retired in Manitoba in 2002. He joined the Mayo Health Care System in Owatonna, Minnesota in 2002 and worked for them for another eight years. He has been fully retired since 2011.

He lives in Mesa, Arizona with his wife Frances, a nurse whom he met while a medical student at the University of Manitoba. He has two daughters, two sons-in-law and two grandchildren.

Acknowledgments

When I look back to where I came from, a Mennonite kid from a poor family with no family role models in academia, I have to give recognition where credit is due.

*My mother would be first. She was a smart woman from a good family.

*Second, would be my religious awakening at an early time in my life, wanting to make a difference and serve my fellow-man. To me the practice of medicine is a calling.

*Third, would be a constant flow of wonderful teachers, starting with Miss Winters in grade school, to my high school teachers and high school principal. The Winkler Collegiate Institute rightfully boasts a marvelous record of success in education.

*Fourth, I will never be able to express sufficient gratitude to Dr. John H. Hildes, my mentor in medical school and dear friend.

Others

During my 38 years in practice in Canada, I had the privilege of working with extraordinary people.

Firstly, I would like to thank Ms. Brenda Picklyk, my office manager for over 30 years in Winnipeg. Due to her ability and loyal service to me and my patients, my office ran smoothly and efficiently until I retired in 2002. I have only praise for the ward and operating room nurses with whom I worked at St. Boniface General Hospital and the Concordia Hospital. I would like to thank the late Professor Ernest Ramsey, who worked with me a few years in private practice, and later became one of Canada's most distinguished urologists. I would particularly like to thank Dr. Barry Caplan, a steadfast friend and associate for 38 years. Other colleagues I am grateful for are the late Dr. Ian MacLeod (my practice partner for over 20 years), Dr. Cliff Smythe, Dr. Wayne Paquin, Dr. Allan Decter, Dr. Bob Yong, Dr. Ross MacMahon, Dr. Martin Rifkin, Dr. Michael Segall and Dr. Grahame Glezerson.

I thank Mr. Sheldon Bowles, Dr. Robert Fulton and Ms. Alexandra Lamont for their feedback on the manuscript. I am grateful for the manuscript review by Ms. Devan Towers of Taylor McCaffrey, LLP.

I would be remiss if I did not acknowledge the love and support of my dear wife Frances who kept things together at home and worked in my office as a nurse for over 20 years.

I would like to thank Ms. Leona M. Krahn whose hard work editing this manuscript was invaluable to me.

Lastly, I owe everything to the country that gave me such enormous opportunity and success. I am a very proud and grateful Canadian.

Chapter 1:
How Medicare Began in Canada

When I was a young medical student in the mid-1950s, there was no such thing as universal healthcare insurance in Canada.

Universal hospital insurance was introduced in 1957 within a free-enterprise framework. Hospitals were owned and managed by church groups, non-profit organizations, municipalities and private corporations. Government insurance paid all the charges. I thought this was a wonderful system. This, more than anything else, besides family connections, enticed me to come back to Canada after my postgraduate training in the US.

Hospitals competed aggressively for competent medical staff. For example, when I returned to Winnipeg from New York City in 1964, my training and qualifications were in great demand. All seven Winnipeg hospitals offered me a staff appointment. There was no shortage of medical specialists in Winnipeg.

Competition for patients kept costs down. Hospitals worked tirelessly to improve the quality of care. Wait lists for admission were unheard of and government monitors made certain discharge delays were justified.

The modus operandi was to eliminate waste, strive for efficiency and excellence. If an untoward event delayed the operating room schedule in the afternoon the surgeon was strongly encouraged to do the case afterhours.

The Administration of the hospital was lean, comprising of a few hired administrators housed in one or two offices in some corner of the hospital and a volunteer Board.

The Board consisted of prominent executives from the business community, church leaders and eminent practicing physicians currently on staff at the hospital. At least half of the Board members were physicians.

Medical teaching was a priority in the teaching hospitals. Experienced busy private physicians did the teaching pro bono. They were recruited by the medical school because of their exemplary standards of medical care. The doctors did this as a reward for the privilege of imparting knowledge and to gain access to the better facilities available in a large teaching hospital.

The standard of care in Winnipeg rivaled the best available anywhere else on the planet. Most of the clinical teachers were trained at prestigious international centers of excellence. There were two big clinics in town that sought to rival the famous Mayo Clinic in the US in professional acumen.

This was a perfect example of social health insurance.

Medical Insurance

By the late 1960s, 85% of the population had voluntarily purchased private medical insurance. There were a number of healthcare insurance companies offering medical coverage, but Manitoba Medical Service (MMS) had the lion's share of the business.

Doctors usually accepted the MMS remittance as payment in full. The doctor could extra-bill if he so desired. However, the extra-billing could be appealed to a Fee Review Committee established by the licensing body. The fee could be deemed excessive by them because of overbilling or the patient's insecure financial status and inability to pay. The decision of the Fee Review Committee was binding. The findings were published by the licensing body. Because of the concern about damaging publicity overcharging was virtually unheard of.

Does Canada Have Socialized Medicine?

There are many who would argue that Canada does not have socialized medicine, they have a single-payer social health insurance system. They will point to the fact the majority of doctors are funded on a fee-for-service basis. They are not under direct government control. They set their own hours and manage their practices as they see fit. It must be conceded this does not fit the socialized medicine mold. However the numbers of doctors allowed on hospital rosters is completely under government control.

Medical school enrollment is limited by the government. Fees are set by the government and there is no extra-billing permitted. The majority of specialists are by now in-hospital based and they are very much under the control of a government Regional Health Authority – they have a signed contract with them.

Let's agree that medical services are a blend of social health insurance and socialized medicine.

Finally, there can be no argument about it being correctly termed socialized medicine when it comes to the hospital system. Hospitals are completely controlled by the Regional Health Authority (RHA). The RHA decides the number of available beds, the operating budget, the staffing ratios, equipment acquisition, and type of service provided and where the services will be located. Site managers cannot lift a finger without first consulting with the RHA. The RHA reports to the government and is accountable to it.

With the personal home care program, it looks at first like it might be a social health insurance model instead of socialized medicine. It is, in fact, an amalgam of the two systems. The institutions are indeed owned and managed by private corporations or non-profit groups. However, the creation of new facilities or the expansion of existing homes cannot occur without government approval.

Since the government maintains absolute control over the stock of beds in personal care homes it is therefore also responsible for shortages. In addition, government determines funding levels, levels of care, and standards of care, client safety and security. All this sounds like government-management to me.

Prescription pharmacies have remained under private corporate control. This instance is a good example of social health insurance instead of socialized medicine. This is a shining example of what the entire Canadian health care system should look like.

Most of the problems with Canadian Medicare are concentrated in the hospital sector and the personal care homes – the fully socialized segments.

Advent of Government-Managed Care (Socialized Medicine)

In 1969, a Manitoba provincial election resulted in a far left-leaning government for eight years. It was within this big-government era that drastic restructuring of the healthcare delivery system occurred. In order to stay within a fixed healthcare budget it was deemed necessary to assert complete control over expenditures and adopt government-managed care, at least in the hospital and personal care home sectors of the healthcare economy. This meant rationing access to hospital care and personal care homes.

This fulfilled the fifth tenet of Tommy Douglas's paradigm for Medicare. The Federal government demanded public administration as a condition for receiving the 50/50 cost-sharing of provincial healthcare expenditures. The blame for this travesty therefore has to be assigned in the main part to a Liberal government that was in power in Ottawa at the time.

Canada soon enacted laws forbidding the provision of any private healthcare outside the established government-managed framework. The law has since been challenged in the Quebec Superior Court and found to be unconstitutional. In the rest of Canada private healthcare facilities are still deemed illegal.

All other industrialized countries with universal healthcare systems (e.g. Great Britain, Australia, and New Zealand, all of Europe) offer a blend of social healthcare insurance and private payment. In fact, the prohibition of private healthcare availability is found only in three countries, namely North Korea, Cuba and Canada.

Canadian healthcare planners modeled the Canadian healthcare system on the Swedish template. I visited Stockholm in July 1960. I was amazed at the parallels between the Karolynska Hospital in Stockholm with our own hospitals here in Winnipeg. There were summer closures, enormous wait lists and hallway medicine –just as we have it in Canada. Alas, Swedish people are smarter than we are; they have reformed their healthcare system. They have privatized much of their system and the availability of services has improved.

In the US, the Health Maintenance Organizations (HMOs) also function as fixed budget institutions. As in Canada, all healthcare services are treated as an expense. They are now a focus of public ridicule. Public services are subordinated by excessive executive salaries, delays in investigations and medical care, rigid adherence to questionable guidelines, poor treatment and outcomes, loss of freedom of choice and enormous wait lists.

American Medicare Advantage (Part C) plans offer, as an enticement, some additional coverage like some dental care. They are HMOs with a fixed network of providers. This is an intrusion by government into freedom of choice.

However, the HMO system and American Advantage plans are still not a monopoly. You can opt out, unless your employer has an undertaking with the HMO that forbids it.

Sadly, in Canada, there is no opting out. You are stuck with Canadian Medicare, except when you get healthcare services at your own expense outside the country (or in Quebec).

Living under Socialized Medicine

Governments use fixed budgets and punitive measures to exercise absolute authority and restraint over expenditure. There is rigid enforcement of a rationing policy, which exists in an unrelenting form to this day. Any deficits have to be recovered the following year.

All private healthcare facilities, except clinics, were either decommissioned or taken over by the Health Authority. It became illegal for individuals to purchase healthcare services from any private vendors in Canada, even with their own money.

Hospital services are usually understaffed to save money. When there is a shortage of staff because of unanticipated reasons, such as illness, services are cancelled without notice. This happens almost daily. Cancellations result in savings.

Also, in the early 1970s, the funding of the Personal Care Homes (PCH) coverage began under Manitoba Health. The number of

PCH beds is rationed, the supply kept way below demand. There is a two year wait list to get access to a bed.

The cost-driven administrator can conserve money if he creates an under supply of physicians. To a Canadian hospital administrator a good doctor is a dreaded liability. He can attract too many clients and cause a strain on the budget.

Of the 38 residents trained under me, only a half dozen or so ever found employment in Winnipeg. Only 40% of the urology trainees across Canada last year found a Canadian hospital that would give them an appointment. In other specialties it was even worse. In cardiovascular surgery 100% were unable to find a hospital appointment in Canada in 2013. Under government-managed healthcare there is always a shortage of medical manpower in the hospital and a glut of qualified doctors who can't find work.

What we hear in academia these days is very little about clinical excellence but a continuous harangue about education and research. It is incomprehensible to me and others, but in the last years of my Winnipeg experience, the University Head of Surgery was a surgeon who seldom operated.

To me the perfect administrative design of a clinical discipline should be like a tricycle. The big wheel in front should always be clinical excellence. The two back wheels should represent education and research. The tricycle needs all three wheels. But there should never be any uncertainty about which is the biggest wheel.

It is axiomatic, delays due to rationing leads to disease progression and more cost. As the saying goes, "A stitch in time saves nine." Rationing may lead to avoidable mortality.

The system is fatally flawed and the problems are not solvable under a socialist system of management. Some other countries, like Sweden, have abandoned the government-managed approach and reverted to a free-market healthcare economy. Canada and the United Kingdom stand alone with this failed system.

Chapter 2:
Manitoba Health

MANITOBA HEALTH IS A GOVERNMENT AUTHORITY TO MANAGE healthcare services in the province of Manitoba.

The Canadian health care system is intended to be the same across Canada. But since each province and territory has sole jurisdiction over its respective healthcare programming it ended up to be somewhat fragmented. Provincial independence asserted itself by demanding minor service and funding deviations across the country. However, provincial healthcare delivery systems must adhere closely enough to the national delivery model in order to qualify for federal funding. Initially, it was 50 percent of the provincial health care budget. Now it is reduced to around 28%.

In the province of Manitoba, where I practiced, the medical system operates in the following manner:

There is a Minister of Health who is an elected representative in the legislature and a member of Cabinet. There are five regional health authorities (RHAs) - one large one for the whole city of Winnipeg and the Churchill area, the Winnipeg Regional Health Authority (WRHA) and four rural regional health authorities.

The Minister of Health appoints a board of directors for each of these RHAs. Approval by the health authority is necessary for every piece of equipment and every staff appointment. The net result is the government and its agent, the respective RHA, is able to exercise absolute control and modify services as it desires. This is the basis of the term, socialized medicine or, more euphemistically stated, government-managed healthcare.

Politically favored projects can be showered with financial support. Programs that do not fit the ideology of the current government in power can be stripped of sufficient funding.

A fixed annual budget is set for the RHA at the beginning of the fiscal year. As the year progresses and funds are spent, program administrators have to plan carefully to make sure they do not run out of money. There is a balance-sheet with only one income source – a government grant. All the public services are on the expense side. The two columns have to be equal at the end of the fiscal year.

A RHA bordering on another province can engage in some gamesmanship. If clients can be persuaded to go to a referral center in another province the tab gets picked up by the province of Manitoba – thus a saving for the RHA. This can be handy when the closest major medical facility is in the adjacent province, a tad closer than in Manitoba. For example, women in labor often go to the nearest obstetrical unit. If that happens to be in another province it's like money in the bank for the RHA.

Of the six acute care hospitals in Winnipeg, four are faith-based and two are secular. Faith-based community representatives, plus city and provincial government appointees comprise the board of directors in each hospital. Although the majority of the board members share a faith affiliation with the original founders, they also have to comply with the directives of the WRHA board, except in matters of conscience as with abortions. The two secular hospitals in Winnipeg perform elective abortions; none of the faith-based hospitals permit them.

The hospital boards exist out of historical necessity but with virtually no power. The power is all vested with the government through the RHA. Physicians are not represented on Manitoba hospital boards except for a few retired physicians and non-voting members like the president of the medical staff. Physicians are not welcome on hospital boards due to concern their potential personal agendas may mess with board decisions. However, a hospital's only excuse for existence is to provide essential services to sick people. There are few with better understanding of patient needs than medical practitioners and frontline staff. Who would be preferable to voice patients' concerns? Physicians are generally considered to be reasonable and responsible citizens; why can't they be trusted to be full voting members of hospital boards?

Allied Medical Institutions

The Manitoba Medical Association (MMA) is the political lobby for the medical profession in the province. It is also responsible for fee negotiations with the government.

The College of Physicians and Surgeons (CP&S) manages the licensing of medical practitioners. The College is not an academic institution as the name implies, simply a licensing board. The physicians at large elect the members of the board. In addition, the government appoints two board members. This organization functions well, serving and protecting the public interest. The College of Physicians and Surgeons' main mandate is to protect the public from unscrupulous or incompetent medical providers. They have the power to suspend or rescind a physician's right to practice medicine.

The Canadian Medical Protective Agency (CMPA) operates as a medical malpractice insurance body. It is doctor-owned and operated, managed by elected representatives from across the country. This terrific organization has kept a lid on malpractice suits in Canada. If a lawsuit appears legitimate, the goal is to admit guilt and settle as quickly and cheaply as possible. If the lawsuit looks frivolous and unjustified, engage in a fierce defense and spare no cost. Lawyers who specialize in suing doctors work on a contingency basis. They are wasting their time if the suit is unlikely to succeed. Because of the CMPA, physician rates for malpractice insurance in Canada are reasonable and affordable.

Five-Pillar Foundation

According to the 2008-2009 Canada Health Act Annual Report, the Canadian health care system is built around five "pillars" or objectives: universality, accessibility, portability, comprehensiveness, and public administration. This model was formulated in the 1950s by the late Saskatchewan Premier, Tommy Douglas – the "father" of Canadian Medicare.

"Universality" means all citizens' essential healthcare needs should be covered by health insurance. Universality also suggests that every Canadian, without exception, is covered by the plan. Universality is limited to in-hospital procedures. For example, ophthalmologists can do cataract operations in the office and thereby escape some of the governmental controls, such as quotas. The government supplies a fixed quota of intraocular lenses in the hospitals each year. When I was practicing in Manitoba, the annual quota filled up quickly, meaning patients often had to wait for the following year or even two years. (This is how it was 10 years ago anyway. This wait list may have improved since then.) To be without a driver's license, unable to read a newspaper, book or enjoy television for two years is a travesty - way too much for most people.

The government could ban in-office cataract surgery and force it to be done in the hospital and get control over the volume. However, it appears the government could not withstand the intense patient pressure and lobbying by ophthalmologists. Now, a patient can purchase the lens directly from his/her ophthalmologist (not affected by the government quota) and get cataract surgery in a timely manner.

There is a problem when physician fees are not the same from province to province. For example, Quebec's fee schedule is the lowest in Canada. When patients seek care in another province the provider may be reluctant or refuse to treat at a discounted fee. The Quebec insurance plan refuses to pay the higher fees set in other provinces. This is a violation of the Canada Health Act which stipulates that provinces must pay the full medical charges established by the province in question. The concept of universality is not without some glaring shortcomings.

"Accessibility" under the five-pillar model guarantees health insurance coverage with uniform terms and conditions, for all persons. This provision was intended to prevent any co-pay or extra-billing issues. The government has some tolerance for a "facility fee" in private doctors' offices. Whether this facility fee is legal or not is an open question – so far the government has turned a blind eye. At any time, however, the government could impose fines or demand reparation payments from physicians. However, accessibility does not necessarily mean "availability" when shortages/rationing are an issue.

"Portability" describes a smooth and seamless transition, with no interruption, when a resident moves from one province to another.

"Comprehensiveness" means all necessary medical services within a hospital setting are covered.

"Public administration" of health care resources means a not-for-profit public authority, accountable only to the government, has complete control over all policies of every health care institution in the province or territory.

Physician Compensation

Canadian physicians are able to work in private practice on a fee-for-service payment system. The fee schedule is arrived at through provincial medical association and government negotiations.

The physicians in the teaching hospitals are almost all "Geographical Full-Time" (GFT). They are paid on a fee-for-service basis, the same as the rest of the medical fraternity, but on a contract basis. All their operating expenses are initially paid by the hospital - no rent, no employee expenses and free supplies. In return they have to agree to a soft income ceiling. They are asked to return to the University and the hospital a substantial percentage of their overage (in excess of the ceiling). This money is then used to fund new recruits. The conditions written into the contract, such as the ceiling and the repayment ratio, is individualized and kept secret. It is therefore possible two doctors carrying the same work load end up with different levels of net remuneration. So much for equal pay for equal work! There is therefore a powerful disincentive built into these employment contracts. Without any overhead expenses you can loaf through most of your day and easily meet your ceiling. Once you are paying overage, which can be 40 or 50%, you might as well go golfing. It's nice work if you can get it.

There are a few other doctors working in public health, northern communities and government-run community clinics on a straight salary.

Opting-in to Medicare

When Medicare was introduced in Canada in 1969, physicians were invited to "opt-in" to the healthcare payment system. They would then receive a monthly check from the government to compensate them for their patient billings. In exchange, those opted-in were forbidden to bill patients any extra amount.

Doctors could also elect to "opt-out" and the compensation for physician services would then go directly to the patient. The opted-out doctor reserved the right to bill the patient any amount he wanted. The overhead cost of fee collection was absorbed by the extra-billing. Within a couple of years, the government disallowed extra-billing by opted-out physicians. The cost of billing patients and the risk of uncollectible accounts created economic disincentives so harsh that very few physicians opted-out from then on.

I chose to opt-out for most of my professional life in Canada. I opted-out on principle at considerable personal expense. The Manitoba Medical Review Committee (a government committee) monitors patterns of practice on a continual basis. My practice profile was far from typical due to the preponderance of cancer patients I looked after. My unusual practice profile placed me at risk for having my fees seized by the government, as was the case with other physicians. If the checks for medical treatment were sent directly to my patients, who would then pay me directly, provided some security. The government could not garnish my fees if it disliked the way I was practicing. The fees would have to be collected back from hundreds of patients, rather difficult. The government's only option for collection would be through the court system.

Because of the financial challenges surrounding collecting fees from patients, I finally relented and chose to opt-in after almost thirty years of standing firm. There are now no opted-out physicians in Manitoba.

Key Components

Canada's national health care system insures four key areas. Universal hospital coverage began in 1958; physician services coverage and nursing home subsidies were introduced in the early 1970s. Prescription pharmacy care (Pharmacare) in Manitoba was launched about 14 years later.

In addition, there are non-government insurance companies that offer indemnity for services not covered by government programs – private room hospital accommodation, dental care and travel health insurance.

Cost of Managing the WRHA

Tom Brodbeck,[*] casts some light on the costs of running the WRHA. He talks about the eleven vice presidents with salaries ranging from $144,645 to $450, 340. In addition, he writes about the Chief Executive Officers in the various institutions getting fat pay checks and pensions.

There is plenty of evidence of management redundancy. This is expected in any government department. The cost of healthcare administration would likely be less if Manitoba Health was turned into a non-profit model with its own Board of Directors – a single-payer sovereign monopoly funded by premiums. The only direct interaction with government should be that it is subject to government scrutiny and regulation. According to Woolhandler, et. al.[**] the average per capita cost of Canadian Medicare administration is $307, or 16.7% of healthcare expenditures. In the US, it is $1,859 or 31% of healthcare expenditures. The cost of healthcare

---

[*] *Tom Brodbeck, Winnipeg Sun, June 29, 2011.*
[**] *Woolhandler, et. .al. New England Journal of Medicine, Aug. 21, 2003.*

administration in the US appears to be five times as much than it is in Canada. I am therefore an ardent proponent of a single-payer system of social health insurance.

American insurance companies spend large sums of money on advertising, political lobbying, and dealing with fee disputes. With a single-payer none of that is necessary.

Chapter 3:
The Unit Cost of Service

To lower the cost of administration, Manitoba Health decided it was a waste of money to price each item of service individually. Since patient billing had been discontinued, why bother with the expense of unit cost accounting? It was the same across Canada.

The only time the general public gets a glimpse at what the charges are is when an American gets sick in Canada. The charges seem to be completely in line with what it costs in the US. I know of an American patient who spent a week in a Canadian hospital, and the fee was over $140,000. There was no surgery involved. This sounds like a lot to me compared to American prices.

Patients never see a bill or account statement in Canada. They have no idea what individual medical services cost. A comparison of unit cost would allow the public to gauge efficiency and cost-effectiveness. For example, it should be possible to compare the cost of a gall bladder operation between hospitals. Is it two or three times more costly in one hospital than the next? If it costs two times as much in a teaching hospital than a community hospital, why are we doing routine elective treatments in the teaching hospital?

The funding process for hospitals is completely opaque and politicized. Legislators with political clout are intent on bringing home the bacon. They shower their constituents with healthcare industry favors to garner their votes. There is no way of finding out how cost-effective these projects are. For example, there is a white elephant called a Birth Center to satisfy a midwifery lobby. What is the unit cost of a birthing course at the Birth Center compared to a hospital or home delivery? The public should judge if it is worth the extra cost at taxpayer's expense. There are QuickCare clinics in Winnipeg, staffed by salaried nurse practitioners (NP). The budget of the clinics has been published. One clinic has a budget of $800,000. No family doctor's office would have a budget anywhere close to that. They seem to cost more than doctor's offices do.

What is the unit cost of care in these clinics? How does it compare to physician fees? Should care by nurses cost more than physician care?

Mind you, I am not opposed to nurse practitioners. In the US I worked with many of them. They are very common at the Mayo Clinic. However, nurse practitioners bill insurance at 85% of the fee paid to physicians, using the same fee schedule.

Chapter 4:
Scarcity and Rationing

Most Canadians think the rationing of healthcare services occurs in only a few select areas, such as joint prostheses, intraocular lenses after cataract surgery and hardly anywhere else. Let's examine this presupposition more closely.

Fixed Budgets

The budget is set for an institution or program by Manitoba Health at the beginning of the fiscal year, similar to a school board budget. There is no other source of income. If there is a deficit it has to be recovered the following year by curtailment of services. Administrators are seldom known to enjoy a surplus, for understandable reasons. It would be clawed back the following year.

Hence every service to a patient in the hospital, every laboratory test and X-ray, has to be treated as an expense. To stay within the annual budget, you must either limit the volume of service (cause scarcity) or dilute the quality of care. A successful administrator's role is to create an institution inefficient enough that he does not run out of money before the end of the fiscal year.

Under social health insurance, an administrator would take great care to keep the cost of production (the unit cost) as low as possible and still retain customer satisfaction. Under socialized medicine, with a fixed budget and no other source of income, the successful hospital administrator is intent on limiting volume and not so worried about the unit cost, or client gratification. It is the exact opposite.

Socialized medicine succeeds in turning the concept of public service upside down. Whereas in social health insurance the client is a source of income and must be carefully nurtured and gratified, with socialized medicine the client is viewed as a dreaded cost.

Efficiency is not the goal. There is only one objective and that is to stay within budget. To accomplish this you do whatever it takes, e.g. turn patients away, dilute services, use inferior or antiquated equipment, limit the number of providers, close beds, curtail overtime, provide insufficient staff and create wait lists for investigations and treatments. Remember, an extra day or two in the hospital for an inpatient not receiving expensive care is money saved.

Fixed budgets lead to scarcity. Scarcity leads to restriction of services (rationing). Rationing leads to inefficiency, waste, and long wait lists and unavailability.

The original premise for the fixed budget notion was to stop the soaring cost of healthcare in Canada. Whether this has been accomplished is debatable. That it has led to the longest wait lists for elective and urgent medical care in the industrialized world is a sad consequence. The belief such long wait lists do not contribute to undue suffering, morbidity and even avoidable fatal outcomes are simple, childlike wishful notions.

What is needed in Canada is an Aleksandr Solzenitzen to raise awareness of the inefficiency of the Canadian healthcare system and the unnecessary human suffering that is underreported by the public media.

Mr. Solzenitzen in his three-volume Gulag Archipelago is famous for exposing the existence and dire conditions in the penal colonies in Siberia during the time of the Soviet Union.

Holiday Bed Closures

One way of keeping patients out of the hospital and saving money is to close one-third of the hospital beds for up to three months a year. How else can the administrator stay within budget? (Those who learn about this hospital administration practice for the first time can't believe this really happens.)

When I was there, there was a partial bed closure (30 percent) for around six weeks in July and August, presumably so staff could enjoy a long summer holiday. There was also a one-week partial closure (also 30 percent) running in conjunction with each of the national holidays. This included New Year's day, Easter, Victoria Day in May, Labor Day in September, Thanksgiving in October, Remembrance Day in November, Christmas and even school breaks in February. Major elective surgeries were halted at least three days before each of these holidays, so that one- third of hospital beds could be closed. All these closures add up to more than three months a year.

Since acute hospital beds are scarce for three months a year, elective sick patients just have to wait.

There are always going to be patients so sick they can't wait. Even though there are hundreds of unused beds upstairs, these unlucky souls languish for a week or so on gurneys in some hospital corridor. Patients with a heart attack, who stay for a week or so, can spend their entire hospital stay on a gurney in the hall. Meanwhile, there are dozens of unused acute care beds upstairs.

Consider how wasteful this bed closure must be. The hospital infrastructure is designed for 100% occupancy. For three months a year one third of the hospital beds are unused. There may be some savings due to staff lay-offs, but of temporary staff only. Since no employee takes a three month holiday each year, many are underutilized for weeks on end each year. That is money that is surely squandered. The cost of financing and depreciation of expensive equipment continues unabated.

The savings don't even amount to much. One year when I was on the hospital board as an ex- officio member. We were told by the administrator of the 132 bed community hospital the saving during the summer months amounted to a mere $160,000. With all this misery the amount saved is no more than what the hospital would normally spend in just a few days.

Deficits in any given year have to be made up the following year. *CBC News Edmonton*[*] in 2013 reported all elective surgeries would be canceled in all Edmonton hospitals for 20 days because of a deficit the previous year. In addition, overtime in the Edmonton hospital operating rooms would be seriously curtailed. (Operating rooms are always a favorite target for cut-backs because this is the most expensive area in any general hospital.)

You really need to hold your nose when you read stuff like this.

Warehousing Patients

Another favorite tactic to reduce cost involves blocking acute care bed usage by warehousing long-stay chronic patients on the wards intended for acute care, rendering beds unavailable for more pricy acute care admissions.

---

* *CBC News, Edmonton, January 30, 2013*

Five percent of all Manitoba hospital admissions become long-stay chronic care patients.* These are patients admitted with an acute illness and then cannot be sent home because their general health conditions are too unstable. Within this group, those with a medical diagnosis stayed an average length of 159 days in the hospital and those with a surgical diagnosis, 208 days. The time was computed from the day the patient was paneled.

The paneling process did not begin until the patient had been in the hospital for at least 30 days. It could take up to 90 days to do the assessment. It is necessary to add all this time to the numbers cited in the previous paragraph to get the picture. Many patients stayed in the hospital for over a year. The report goes on to state 39 percent of Winnipeg hospital acute care beds were occupied by patients no longer able to cope at home but not requiring hospital care. (You read it correctly – 39 percent of beds!) Obviously, hospitals had no great desire to part with these patients.

Not only were these occupants blocking acute care patient admissions, they were also not receiving appropriate care. They were not accessing memory-loss programming, getting socializing opportunities and other supports usually available in a personal care home.

The hospital administrator operates on the premise that lodgers cost little more than room and board. Acute care patients, on the other hand, might cost thousands of dollars a day.

According to a publication written by Marcy Cohen of the Fraser Institute,** the daily cost of warehousing a senior in an acute care bed ranges from $825 to $1,968 a day in BC. This figure is arrived at by dividing the annual budget by patient days in the hospital. Infrastructure costs necessary for a hospital are not needed for clients just getting room and board. These resources are wasted

---

*   *Manitoba Center for Health Policy Report, 2,000.*
**   *Caring for BC's Aging Population, Fraser Institute, July 2012.*

when patients only receive room and board. The cost of a personal home care home bed is around $200 a day. For every patient warehoused in an acute care bed in the hospital, at least a half-dozen infirm elderly could be accommodated in a personal care home at the same cost.

Overtime in the Operating Room

The operating room has the biggest discretionary budget in the hospital. If an administrator wants to rein-in costs this is the area that interests him before anywhere else.

The administrator of a Canadian hospital cannot afford to allow much overtime in the operating room. The negotiated labor contract with the nurses' union stipulates if operating room nurses work more than 15 minutes overtime they have to be paid a minimum of four hours at an overtime rate of pay. Working with a fixed annual budget, this is not affordable. And for the patient to wait for the next operating day a week later costs the hospital little more than three square meals a day. Patients stay in the hospital because they do not want to risk losing their place in the queue. This is where there is a stark difference between a government-managed healthcare economy and a market-driven system. In a profit motivated system this would never be tolerated.

In my experience, American healthcare industry unions do not possess the clout that Canadian unions do. Most healthcare institutions, including the Mayo Clinic, do not even have a healthcare union. No American hospital administrator would ever enter into an agreement where they would pay an employee for four hours of work when they only worked sixteen minutes of overtime.

Secondly, every healthcare institution in the United States is aware of what the competition is doing across town. Poor public relations are quickly translated into monetary penalties.

Thirdly, to house a patient for a whole week, offering only room and board, while waiting for the surgeon's next surgery date would be far too expensive in a market-driven institution. Look at all the income that is missed while the hospital bed is used for hostel purposes only. The business depends on fee-for-service income to flourish economically.

To give an example, on my surgery day at a Mayo Clinic hospital one afternoon I had one more elective operation to perform at three o'clock in the afternoon. There was a crash on the highway and a number of seriously injured patients were admitted requiring immediate surgery. My patient was sent back to the ward and I was asked to remain on standby. At 11:30 pm. my phone rang asking me to come in to do the preplanned surgery. They did what they could to accommodate the patient.

In Canada, my cancer of the prostate surgery cases usually took about three hours of surgery time. I would plan to do two cases back to back every Thursday. Many things can delay the first case. For example, a super-slow anesthesiologist can take two or three times longer than usual to put the patient to sleep. There can be problems with the first surgery and more time taken. I would get away with being 15 minutes overtime, but not 20 or 30. Then the second surgery would always be canceled.

These patients were completely prepped for surgery. That costs real money. Multiple units of blood had already been shipped to the hospital.

Preoperative anxiety levels are always very high in patients before major surgery – sometimes overwhelming. For example, I had a patient who died in the elevator on the way to the operating room.

Since he appeared, otherwise, perfectly healthy it was concluded that it was a panic attack that killed him. To go through all this anxiety and then get canceled at the last moment for a frivolous reason is beyond the bounds of morality. In Canadian hospitals it happens all the time.

There is also the impact on the rest of the family to be considered. Many have traveled from out of town and are greatly inconvenienced. They may have booked a room in a hotel. There is no compensation for these extra expenses. Looking back at this now, many years later, I still feel queasy about this. Part of the surgeon's job is to explain to patients the reason for the cancellation (not enough time) and shoulder the blame for it. The family naturally assumes that the surgeon must have mismanaged something. That it was caused by administrative wrongdoing never occurs to them.

Beyond regulation, there is no other fitting role for the government in hospital management.

Job Actions

Job actions, such as strikes and a union "work to rule", are prevalent in the Canadian hospital system. Any threat of a strike results in a drastic reduction of admissions so that beds can be closed in preparation - more than half of a hospital's beds. Many different unions bargain with hospital administration, all independent of each other. They negotiate at different times. Strikes can last for four weeks or longer.

A research paper by Stabler and others,[*] analyzes a four week province-wide nurses' strike in Alberta in 1982. The investigators found that there was no loss of life during the strike that could be attributed to the job action by the nurses. The full range of emergency

---

[*] *Stabler, et. al., Canadian Medical Journal, August, 1984.*

services was maintained during the strike period. Elective surgeries, including cancer surgery, were all discontinued during the duration of the strike. The effects of pain or inconvenience to the patients were not included in the study. Also, there was no mention of the possible ultimate consequences of delaying the treatment. A rapidly progressing cancer can metastasize if treatment is delayed for a month. Urgent patients who die on the wait list outside the hospital would not be counted.

When 57% of the acute care beds are closed for a month because of a strike the hospital enjoys major savings. The Chief Financial Officer of the hospital may think that a long strike is a godsend.

If the goal of the striking employees is to inflict damage to the institution it is obvious they are missing their target. The closure results in enormous savings. The people who suffer from a prolonged strike are the general public and the strikers themselves. By union agreement, the hospital cannot lay-off full-time employees who are not on strike. The hospital ends up paying hundreds of underutilized staff. This is wasted money. Temporary employees, on the other hand, can be laid off without compensation. Therefore, hospitals in Canada offer new nursing and health technology graduates only part-time employment for as long as possible. I have a nephew, a laboratory technician, who has worked for a hospital for five years and is still a temporary employee. The status of "temporary" robs them of benefits and protection. These young people are mute victims of a government-managed health care system. Strikes are settled when the government can no longer placate public demand. The unions usually get almost everything they have requested.

The public interest deserves a more moderate process than a strike to settle a labor dispute in a hospital. For the strikers, finding a better weapon than a strike could be to their advantage as well.

Shortage of Equipment

According to the Fraser Institute,[*] Canada still lags far behind most other countries in the availability of medical equipment. Here are some of the rankings:

CT scanners – 16th out of 23 countries
MRI – 14th out of 22 countries
PET scanners – 11th out of 20 countries
Lithotripters – 15th out of 17 countries

There is a huge reluctance on the part of a government-managed economy to adequately supply funding to furnish enough medical infrastructure. Enhanced efficiency in investigation might result in more volume and put more stress on the fiscal budget. However, this is a highly questionable thesis. Disease is progressive and a delay of many weeks or even months always creates a much more expensive treatment protocols and even avoidable deaths. Long wait lists and delayed treatment have never saved a penny.

According to the above-mentioned 2012 report, the average wait period for a CT scan across Canada is 3.7 weeks, for MRI 8.4 weeks and for Ultrasound 3.7 weeks. CIHI,[**] a government-funded data collector, confirms these troubling wait times. In Manitoba, in 2012, the wait time for a CT scan was 35 days and for MRI was 119 days. In Nova Scotia, the wait time for CT scans was 74 days and for MRI 135 days. In Alberta the wait time for CT scan was 37 days, but for MRI 235 days.

Moreover, the acquisition of medical infrastructure is riddled with politics. The most graphic example of the politicization of medical equipment procurement occurred in Ontario. According to a debate

---

[*]   *Fraser Institute, April 12, 2012.*
[**] *CIHI Report on Wait Times in Canada, 2012.*

in the Ontario legislature, *Hansard*,* a lithotripter had been purchased with private money to be located in Hamilton. The Ontario government had decided, for political reasons, that a lithotripter should be located only in Toronto and in London, Ontario. The Toronto lithotripter could only handle 1,100 patients a year and there was a demand for 5,000 patients to be treated. Meanwhile, Hamilton patients were sent to Buffalo, NY, where the cost of treatment was twice as much as in Toronto.

Permission was never granted and the machine sat idle in storage until they were able to get rid of it – never used.

Age-Related Guidelines

A friend of mine, a retired, otherwise healthy physician, needed a hip replacement at the age of 94. His orthopedic surgeon told him he was too old and could not have the surgery.

He bought his own hip prosthesis and looked for a surgeon to put it in. He found one who was willing. The surgeon discussed the plan with the department heads at the teaching hospital. I was at the meeting and we heartily supported the idea. However, he could not get permission from the administrator of the hospital. It was doubtless vetoed by the WRHA. That would have been two-tiered medicine; one level of care for the rich and another for the poor. He lived to 106, meaning he spent the last 12 years of his life in pain and in a wheelchair.

In a truly free society, patients should have access to medical services at any age if deemed medically fit enough. With government-managed health care, the governing policy can limit eligibility for treatment on the basis of age rather than the physical status and life expectancy of the patient.

---

*   *Ontario Hansard, December 6, 1989.*

Canada prohibits the purchasing of health care at your own expense. It should never be illegal to get treatment if you pay for it yourself. Canada is supposed to be a democracy. Canada's Bill of Rights is an off-shoot of the Magna Carta, dated 1215. This limits the power of government and protects the rights of the people. For a thousand years all English commonwealth people have lived under Magna Carta protection. Canadian parliamentarians have evidently never heard of it.

Quotas

In areas where prosthetics are involved quotas are easy to impose. The temptation seems irresistible. There are quotas for lenses in cataract surgery and for artificial joints. This is still going on in late 2014. For example, an effective and efficient joint replacement program at the Concordia Hospital in Winnipeg was told by the WRHA in September, 2014 to curtail such surgeries. They were exceeding their quota.

But there are other forms of rationing. For instance, the best chemotherapy drugs are not always available because of cost and, as a result, fewer cancer patients survive their disease. If screening for cancer is not allowed, avoidable deaths due to cancer go up.

In early February, 2014, I was at a book signing in Phoenix, AZ., where I met a very robust looking gentleman in his 60's who was a recent immigrant to the US from Calgary, AB. He had two bone marrow transplants in Canada for a bone marrow malignancy and needed a third one. He was told in Canada they were rationed and two was all they allowed. He moved to the US in November, 2013. The Affordable Care Act (Obamacare) kicked in on January 1, 2014. He made an appointment and received a bone marrow transplant in Phoenix within two weeks at minimal cost to him. There was no wait period. Under Obamacare there are no exclusions due to preexisting conditions. Rationing in Canada can kill people who are relatively young and still have the prospect of many years of good health.

Rationing is also seen in the issuance of medical supplies. For example, I have a friend who died recently in Winnipeg from a pulmonary embolus eight days after radical cancer surgery. He was only 67 years old and otherwise in perfect health. Pneumatic compression stockings are known to prevent blood clots from forming in the legs during and immediately after major surgery. These blood clots can migrate to the lungs and cause sudden death. The appliances cost about $500. In the US, pneumatic compression stockings after surgery are considered mandatory. I had a shoulder replacement in Scottsdale and spent one night in the hospital. Compression stockings were used. Apparently, in Canada, they are not used routinely because they cost too much. Could this death be attributed to a penny-pinching government-managed health care system?

There is another insidious form of rationing. In Manitoba the government has a Medical Review Committee that keeps a spread sheet documenting everything that a physician orders. In my own practice I was found to be an outlier (not average) because of the high percentage of patients in my practice with prostate cancer. Since I deviated significantly from the norm I had to appear before the committee to explain myself. Doctors can be subject to sanctions if they are outside the norm and do not shape up. In my case, they accepted my explanation and I was forgiven.

Many physicians who ignore government guidelines, or are otherwise outside the norm (outliers), can leave a Medical Review Committee facing enormous penalties. The most extreme example of rationing I have heard about exists in Ontario. According to the *Ottawa Sun,* June 10, 2012, bureaucrats in the Ontario Ministry of Health will henceforth decide whether tests ordered by doctors are "medically necessary". If tests have been done without prior government approval, the physician may be asked to pay for them himself.

This puts someone who has never examined the patient between the doctor and the sick person. Who should the invalid trust more, his doctor or some government character he has never met?

My libertarian instincts are offended by the intrusion of the government into a personal doctor/patient relationships involving life or death. How can a doctor keep the best interests of the patient as his highest priority when he is constantly being second-guessed, often by somebody with only a high school diploma?

The upshot of all this is the doctor lives in constant fear the government might pounce on him for over-servicing his patients. He could be vilified in public because sanctions against doctors are zealously reported in the media. Doctors in Canada survive by keeping their heads down and avoid the government flak that is flying all around them. It is best not to step out of line and stay safe. Don't order the test that a Government guideline may forbid. The patient should always come first. But under socialized medicine government directives come first. The government people tell you what is best practice. The doctor is just a small peon quietly following rules.

Chapter 5:
Wait List

THE PUBLIC IS LED TO BELIEVE THE WAIT LISTS IN CANADA ARE NO more than an inconvenience. Pain and suffering don't count. If there are avoidable deaths resulting from long wait lists and cancellations, nobody knows of any. Furthermore, no one is interested in finding out.

The scientific community publishes research comparing longevity and survival based on broad surveys of clustered populations, e.g. breast cancer survival. This kind of research is virtually useless and should be disregarded. The results are tainted by lead-time bias if screening is employed and by unrelated factors such as better nutrition and support.

The research that would be acceptable would be based on internationally recognized benchmarks and examining outcomes based on survival of those that meet the benchmark and those that don't. For example, do those with a heart attack and get stented in less than 90 minutes fare better than those who don't?

How serious is the problem with wait lists for urgent surgery in Winnipeg? Another study[*] examined the date of the patient's last

---

[*] *Manitoba Center for Health Policy, 2007.*

visit with his/her surgeon and the subsequent date of surgery. This study spanned the years 1999 to 2004. The resultant waiting times were as follows:

Coronary artery bypass – 41 days
Heart valve replacement – 65 days
Cataract surgery – 16 weeks
Gallbladder removal, breast tumor removal, carotid endarterectomy – 18 to 42 days
Varicose vein repair – 93 days
Carpal tunnel – 58 days
Prostate surgery (non-cancerous) - 38 days
Tonsillectomy – 70 days
Hip replacement – 28 weeks
Knee replacement - 31 weeks

I am surprised the wait periods were not much longer. During the last years of my Winnipeg practice, my patients with prostate cancer had to wait four months for surgery. Out of a sense of desperation, I used to prescribe hormone therapy to these patients in an attempt to slow down their cancer while they were waiting.

There is a major flaw in the methodology of this study. It assumes that the treatment plan was formulated at the time of the last visit with the surgeon. According to them this was when the wait period began.

There has to be a pre-operative medical assessment done within one month of the surgery. This includes a physical examination, a list of current medications, blood work, a chest X-ray, and a heart tracing. The hospital demands all of this be done within four weeks of the surgery to ensure that the patient is physically fit for an operation. The last office visit may have nothing to do with the wait list. Many surgeons do their own physicals. This would make it appear that patients waited less than a month. It is therefore impossible to authenticate these data. However, assuredly the average wait time would be much longer.

The only true way to ascertain accurate wait list periods would be to directly ask the patients or the front line caregivers, such as the surgeons. It appears they were not consulted for this study. At least, I wasn't. A wait list should be the time from the first symptom to the time of treatment. This would include the time it takes to see the primary physician, the specialist and the wait to get the tests done. This study ignores all of that. To get an accurate picture of the wait time at least another two or three months should be added to all the times listed above.

Another aspect of the wait list problem that should be considered in Canada is the effect that this has on Canada's gross national product. Productivity is lost when workers sit at home waiting to be treated. These losses could amount to billions of dollars a year.

It is the long wait lists seen with cancer patients that are the most worrisome. The oncologists are the ones who see the result of the long wait list. They are front-row witnesses to the morbidity and avoidable death toll that ensues from waiting too long. There are probably hundreds of avoidable cancer deaths each year due to the long wait lists for medical appointments, investigations and treatment. The government-managed healthcare system has plenty of skeletons in its closet.

In the US, we have seen congressional hearings into avoidable deaths in the VA hospital system. Witnesses are summoned to testify under oath. That is what is needed in Canada. Oncologists in Canada should tell us, under witness protection, how they feel about the long wait lists to see a doctor, the investigations and treatments.

Canadians view long wait lists for elective and urgent care with complacency. They contend it doesn't matter if a person waits for a year or two for a new hip or a new knee. There is support for this opinion in the medical journals. Outcomes are reported no worse in Canada than in other industrialized countries.

There is something delusional going on here. As Mark Twain put it, "Facts are stubborn things, statistics are pliable." It depends on what is being measured. The best way to gauge results is to use agreed to bench-marks and measure the number of times they are met and whether it makes any difference.

Wait List for Emergency Patients

Canadians have the perception that when it counts, when it is really serious, the treatment is usually timely and of superior quality. As they say, "Ignorance is bliss". Canadians don't have a clue what happens when there is a medical emergency. Here wait lists have to be measured in minutes, not weeks or months. Early stenting of a coronary artery may make the difference between becoming a cardiac cripple and a perfectly healthy person. These are the wait times that matter the most. This matters far more than the wait periods for elective healthcare.

The casual observer, or lay person, does not appreciate critical moments are being lost. I was discussing this with a retired physician friend of mine the other day. His wife recently had a heart attack. I asked him how long it took to get stented in Winnipeg's "heart hospital". You guessed it – it took two days because it happened on a weekend. He thought the care had been terrific.

It is impossible to do a proper controlled study of morbidity and mortality of delays and cancellations of emergency cases. They would have to separate patients into a study group and a control group and compare complications and mortality. Patients in the placebo group might fare much worse, resulting in legal and moral questions asked. Who would volunteer to be in the placebo group?

However, you can study the number of patients treated within the time-frame of an internationally agreed to benchmark. You can then determine if the outcome differs between the two groups. This should be fertile area for academic research. According to MedlinePlus (US National Library of Medicine) stent placement should happen within 90 minutes of the onset of a heart attack. The time is calculated from arrival at the ER to the time it takes for the guidewire to pass through the blockage in the coronary artery. The treatment of a stroke involves a pretreatment CT scan to differentiate a major vessel occlusion from a hemorrhage. The guideline stipulates anticoagulation should start within 90 minutes.

Last minute cancellations of urgent cases are not a rare event in Winnipeg. On April 15, 2010,* it was reported in 2009 there were 262 last-minute heart surgery cancellations in Manitoba, including 43 in the month of December alone. These figures were confirmed by the Manitoba Minister of Health. A WRHA spokeswoman also confirmed the CBC finding.

On January 21, 2015, an outside study of Winnipeg's Cardiac Science Program showed there had been 120 cancellations in 2013. The heart program had asked permission to start heart transplants in Winnipeg. Because of this appalling record of delays and cancellations, approval for the program was denied. In addition, there were 4,000 patients on the wait list for an echocardiogram, an essential test in the investigation of heart function.

Consider the plight of a 62 year old man with highly unstable angina, admitted for a coronary artery bypass grafting procedure (CABG) in a hospital that specializes in heart disease in Manitoba. He had been on the waiting list outside the hospital as an extremely urgent patient for over a month. He was finally scheduled for 1 pm on a certain day. Unfortunately, after getting all psyched up, and having

---

* *CBC News Manitoba, April 15, 2010.*

his family with him, it did not happen. The surgery was cancelled at the last moment because there was no ICU bed available. However, they promised, he would be operated on the following week.

Meanwhile, of course, he was occupying an acute care bed without receiving any treatment. Parenthetically, the hospital was OK with that. They were 'saving' thousands of dollars when the bed was blocked for acute care.

The same thing happened the next week – again cancelled at the last moment for the same reason. He died a few days later without ever getting the life-saving surgery.

I would like to relate the true story of two physicians who had a severe heart attack at about the same time in 2006. One was in Minnesota, 38 miles from a tertiary center and the other in Manitoba, 100 miles from the nearest heart hospital.

In the Minnesota case, the physician collapsed at home and was transported to the Emergency Department. Two things happened within the first five minutes. A helicopter was ordered and massive doses of anticoagulants were given. In exactly 56 minutes the patient arrived on the roof of the tertiary hospital and surgery was begun. The operating room team was already fully assembled, gowned and ready to go. The doctor got through this with no permanent heart damage.

In the other case, the doctor collapsed at home while mowing the lawn. The wife called "911" and the emergency medical team responded quickly. During the trip to Winnipeg by ambulance, my doctor friend and the technician, riding in the back of the ambulance, tried the paddles for the electro-shock machine but they did not fit. He was taken to the wrong hospital in Winnipeg. He finally got to the right place and was put on the wait list for stent placement. This was done two days later.

Both doctors survived. The WRHA would argue it made no difference.

The Minnesota doctor went back to work full-time. The Manitoba doctor was left a cardiac cripple and retired. However, there is no scientific basis to contend the delay made the difference. When proof is not obtainable you have to rely on common sense.

I asked a Winnipeg interventional physician, "How often does the "heart hospital" in Winnipeg meet an internationally agreed to 90 minute bench-mark for stenting in heart attacks and strokes?"

He replied, "I really don't know. I have never heard of such a bench-mark."

"That's strange," I said. "In the US, you can google any hospital offering interventional cardiology and the accreditation agency will document if they meet the benchmarks."

Given that in an emergency minutes count, I suspect the standard of critical healthcare in Canada is just as deplorable as is the status of elective care. We need Canadian data on how long it takes a patient to get from the door of the Emergency Department to the operating room. Are benchmarks used and are they met?

Chapter 6:
Quality Controls

BY NOW THE READER MUST HAVE GATHERED MY BIGGEST CONCERN about a government-managed healthcare system is the lack of independent oversight and regulation. Management and oversight do not belong in the same office together. There is too great a temptation to cover-up or gloss-over any mistakes.

Moreover, the lay public is not qualified to judge the quality of the treatment they are receiving. Independent qualified analysts with the know-how to judge whether it is good or bad should always hover in the background. Such evaluations should become part of the public record.

In the US, hospitals are regulated by the Joint Commission on Accreditation (JCACHO). There are regular detailed inspections. The auditors focus on the width of corridors, the equipment in the operating rooms, and the cleanliness of patient's rooms. They also look at standards of patient care. You can google the JCACHO website and see if your local hospital meets treatment benchmarks.

When there is a complaint the JCACHO team does an immediate audit. Lapses in performance should always be investigated and dealt with by an impartial third party.

Compliance with benchmarks is mandatory if accreditation is expected. With a heart attack the time to the operating room should be less than 90 minutes. With a stroke it should be the same, 90 minutes to get the CT scan and start anticoagulants.

The media and parliamentary opposition play important roles as healthcare policy critics but face limitations due to a lack of unbiased, nonpartisan studies and healthcare databases. In the United States, private hospitals and other healthcare institutions are all subject to scrutiny by third-party inspectors.

For example, the *Winnipeg Free Press*, May 15, 2010, shared the account of an investigation into the death of a 19-year-old woman in 2006. She died of a massive hemorrhage from an injured aorta following a serious motor vehicle accident in rural Manitoba.

According to the article, when she arrived at the trauma center during the night, it was soon discovered, as a result of a chest CT scan, there was a five centimeter aortic injury threatening to burst at any moment. Eventually, the aorta ruptured and she quickly bled to death. This injury to the aorta was known about for at least four hours before she died. Nothing was done to repair it.

A WRHA investigation ensued, but it took nearly four years for the report to be released. The ultimate conclusion – "the doctors gave conflicting stories". To me this looks like a political "white-wash."

What kind of useless investigation comes up with such a flimsy conclusion? A worthless report like that could have been tendered within ten minutes. Here was an obvious breach of public safety that was covered up. Nothing should bother the public more than the fact there is no one to offer objective criticism within a government-managed healthcare system framework.

Healthcare institutions and their regulators are both branches of the same government.

When an egregious event like this occurs in the police department, the local police department would never head the inquiry. An independent investigator from another city would be brought in to examine the incident. For the WRHA to investigate itself is definitely problematic.

On the other hand, this case sounds like possible medical malpractice. The complaint should never have been politicized by government involvement in the first place. This falls within the purview of the College of Physicians and Surgeons (CP&S). The authority to investigate complaints about physician neglect rests with them and not with the government. Was this case ever reported to the CP&S?

Regulation of hospitals should include assessment of qualifications, equipment standards, mortality and morbidity rates, length of stay, infection rates, and medical records and on and on. However, physician malpractice belongs within the purview of the licensing body, the CP&S.

These inquiries must be done by an impartial investigator. The politicization of physician ability and performance is abhorrent and should be avoided.

Patient Satisfaction Polls

If you live in the US you are bombarded with advertisements from hospitals and clinics soliciting your patronage as a patient. It is a competitive world out there.

To beat the competition in the US, the provider tries very hard to please. To identify weaknesses in performance they use a patient satisfaction questionnaire. Hence, every major institution will poll patients after a service to identify deficiencies. The provider has to keep ahead of the competitor across the street.

When there is a single-payer healthcare system the regulator should do this. This should become the corner-stone of the regulatory edifice.

With socialized medicine there is no competition. The need to worry about ratings does not exist. The patient has nowhere else to go. In the institutions, patients are not a source of income – they actually cost money. It would be better if there were fewer patients. There is no point in trying to boost your popularity. Doctors working for HMOs on salary in the US find that their compensation is usually based on patient satisfaction data. A poor bed-side manner can cost you a raise in pay or a bonus.

During my time with the Mayo Health Care System I found myself compared with about 100 other urologists in my peer group. The information was doubtless valuable to my employers. It was also very useful to me. I appreciated knowing how I ranked in patient satisfaction.

Polling is not the answer. When Gallop did a telephone survey of health care services in the US, Canada and Great Britain in March, 2003 they found patient satisfaction was much higher in the two countries with government-managed care than in the US with private care. In the US it was 6%, in Great Britain 43% and Canada 57%. These surprising results probably reflect the way the question was asked. The question was, "are you satisfied with affordable healthcare in the nation?"

We know from other national polling that 85% of Canadians like their health care system. How much of this approval rating is driven by slanted government news releases? The public needs to have access to fair and balanced analysis and objective commentary from independent sources before they make up their minds. They have to be shown four of the pillars of Tommy Douglas' vision in healthcare would not be weakened by adopting a single-payer social insurance system.

Would the result be the same if there was a patient satisfaction poll of patients who had recently been treated in a Canadian health care facility? That is why we need patient satisfaction exit polling data.

If I designed a Canadian patient satisfaction exit poll I would ask questions like this:

1. Were you satisfied with the care provided?

2. Was there a long wait list for tests or treatments?

3. Was there screening for cancer?

4. Was your surgery canceled at the last minute?

5. Was the provider courteous and friendly?

6. Did the provider explain things adequately so you could understand?

7. Did the provider offer alternative treatments?

8. Did the provider offer referral for a second opinion?

9. Did the provider give you a reminder a day or two before?

10. Was he thorough in the examination?

11. Was the receptionist friendly and helpful?

12. Was the office clean and orderly?

13. Was the office certified and the certificate posted?

This is just a sample of what a patient satisfaction form in the US looks like.

Explanation of Benefits

The explanation of benefits form is another document Canadians are unfamiliar with.

In the US, after every medical service a document arrives in the mail from the hospital, Medicare and the insurance company listing in detail the services rendered and a detailed breakdown of the fees requested and the compensation granted. The hospital report has three columns, the part paid by Medicare, the part paid by the co-insurance company and the part that is your own responsibility. The insurance company document is essentially the same.

The Medicare report tells you if you should pay the additional amount the provider is charging. The report says in bold letters, "The extra amount charged by the provider does not need to be paid". This is truly amazing! In this case the government is taking good care of you and protecting you from overcharging.

Canadian Medicare Abuses

The Canadian healthcare system authorities maintain physicians should not be owners of medical equipment such as ultrasound machines. This could result in over prescribing because of self-referral. They may have a point; there is a definite risk of this happening. A deductible or co-pay would put a stop to this.

Patient's convenience is enhanced by having the investigative equipment on-site. Wait times are much shorter. The practicing physician is the boss and when he wants it now, he gets it immediately.

To be sure, free healthcare can lead to frivolous patient requests. Doctors' offices are often packed with people seeking mild pain killer prescriptions or stuffy nose remedies. These are all readily available "over the counter" at the local pharmacy and do not need a doctor visit or prescription. For some, a visit to the doctor adds interest to an otherwise dull day.

A study in Manitoba,* reviewed the records of patients who made more than 67 medical visits a year, or saw more than 12 doctors annually. The worst abuser made 247 visits and saw 71 different doctors in one year!

They applied new restrictions on these patients (28 patients) and saved $165,000.

A study in Quebec,** funded by CIHI, reports that Canadians still reject the idea of a deductible to curb patient abuse.

Data

On April 13, 2013, the Canadian Broadcasting Corporation (CBC) flagship investigative journalism program *the fifth estate* reported it was denied requested information from Canadian hospitals that would allow them to create a national hospital rating system.

The CBC later discovered via Canada's Freedom-of-Information Act provincial and territorial health department officials met and agreed, on a national basis, to deny the CBC the necessary information.

In the United States, all hospitals are owned by non-government entities, except for hospitals owned by the Department of Veterans Affairs (VA), the military, and Indian Affairs. With the exception of these, all hospitals are inspected and certified by an independent agency, the Joint Commission on Accreditation of Hospital Organizations (JCAHO). Nursing homes are inspected by the Centers for Medicare and Medicaid Services (CMS). These are regulators who maintain a searchable database.

---

*   *Canadian Medical Journal, May 1, 1995.*
**   *Health Affairs, May, 2004.*

Journalists mining data from these regulatory agencies in the United States produce helpful hospital ratings, like the annual list of best hospitals in America by the *U.S. News and World Report*.

Patients in both countries are now establishing online data banks themselves via sites like *Rate Your Doctor*.

The Canadian Institute for Health Information (CIHI) collects performance data on Canadian healthcare institutions. CIHI is described as an "independent", not-for-profit corporation. CIHI compares length-of-stay, infection rates, and mortality rates, and so on in all hospitals across Canada.

I am skeptical about CIHI's "independence". According to the CIHI website, all of CIHI expenses are funded by federal, provincial and territorial government sources. It rings plausible that "he who pays the piper calls the tune". CIHI may be just as political as any department of the government – claims of independence notwithstanding.

CIHI in Canada is probably just as good at collecting data as JCAHO in the United States. The difference is that political considerations may dominate its agenda and effectiveness. This slant/bias arguably limits the usefulness of all this information. When it suits the government to provide information in a positive light, then CIHI data is proudly presented. When findings might prove embarrassing to the government, the information window appears to slam shut.

For example, where is the data documenting time to treatment for heart attack and stroke patients? How do these data compare with internationally agreed to benchmarks in other first world countries?

Obviously, Canada is blessed with very skilled government spinmeisters. They tell us that delays in treatment don't compromise outcomes. I don't believe anything the government says. I need to see proof. Maybe Canadians should heed G. K. Chesterton's advice. He said, "Do not be so open-minded that your brains fall out".

It is a pity that analytical reporting of healthcare concerns and astute commentary is so rare in Canada.

Other Data Collections

The Fraser Institute in British Columbia is funded by private industry. They do some excellent independent research and reporting on Canadian healthcare system woes, such as wait times for elective healthcare and shortage of investigative equipment. A great example is their report on the average wait time to see a specialist (19 weeks).*

The Canadian Association of Gastroenterology surveyed bowel specialists across Canada in April 2012. It takes an average of 161 days to see a bowel specialist in Canada from the initial date of referral by the family doctor. In Manitoba, the average wait was 249 days. A similar study in 2008 showed an average wait time of 155 days in Canada and 258 days in Manitoba. The situation is not getting any better.** The study also revealed referrals related to rectal bleeding required an average 82 day wait to see a specialist in Canada (143 days in Manitoba).

Rectal bleeding is widely recognized as one of the first indications of bowel cancer. Due to the wait time, many cases of rectal and colon cancer are surely diagnosed too late. There must be hundreds of avoidable deaths. The Manitoba Minister of Health was asked to comment on this report. She dodged the question, stating she needed to know more about the study methodology. We need to take the politics and the propaganda out of this and get to the facts.

---

*   *Waiting Your Turn, Fraser Institute, 2010.*
** *Winnipeg Free Press, June 20, 2012.*

We need more investigative journalism in Canada. Multiple independent studies should be constantly underway to keep us abreast of Canada's health care status. But accessing accurate data requires the full cooperation by government healthcare agencies and institutions and no stonewalling. Otherwise, we will never know the truth. The public are entitled to key information and it should be freely provided. Government ought to be reminded it is there to serve the public and not stoop to obfuscation and concealment.

Since unvarnished reports on the Canadian healthcare system are so rare we are left to rely mostly on rumor and anecdotal evidence to measure the system's shortcoming.

The Cost of Quality

When you visit a private Canadian clinic you sense immediately that times must be tough. The dated atmosphere in some private clinics is not just cosmetic. There are also problems with antiquated equipment, overcrowding and obvious staff shortages.

For example, in urology, a specialist can purchase a rigid scope for about $1,000. A flexible scope costs $20,000. There are fine wires in the flexible instrument that break easily and often. The maintenance costs are considerable.

In the last 20 years, since they were first introduced, I always used the flexible scope. I could hook it up to a monitor so everyone in the room, including the patient, could see exactly what I was seeing. I had to have three of them, because one would almost always be out for repair. Also, I had to have two of them on hand at all times because cleaning and sterilization took longer. I lost money on every office cystoscopy. Flexible scopes are much more comfortable for the patient. You can peek around corners, into bladder pockets (diverticuli) and do a more thorough examination.

All Canadian urologists would use flexible scopes if they could afford them. However, a $60 fee for a cystoscopy does not cover the overhead, let alone leave anything to live on. Therefore, it is necessary for the urologist is to use the cheapest instrument available, or do the procedure in a hospital outpatient department. There the instruments and staff are supplied by the hospital at no cost to him. However, this is inconvenient for both the doctor and the patient. It is virtually impossible for an independent practitioner to get treatment privileges. Hospital-based investigations are fraught with dreadfully long wait lists.

Such quandaries are encountered every day in the office of every private practitioner in the country.

The cost in the hospital involves registration, the cost of a recovery room and a host of other ancillary expenses. The hospital cost is easily two or three times more than an office procedure. However, this all comes out of the hospital budget, so what the heck.

When it comes to switching to electronic medical records; that would be an unaffordable stretch – an utterly unthinkable notion! Yesteryear's technology will have to suffice.

The regulators should inspect clinics and make certain that they comply with minimum standards. Chintzy providers should be shut down. The regulators should also pressure the insurer to provide adequate fee reimbursement.

Chapter 7:
Lack of Incentives

INCENTIVES CAN INCREASE BOTH THE EFFICIENCY AND QUALITY OF health care performance. This is why the large HMOs in the US are all turning towards business models with built in incentives. The idea that remuneration should be linked to seniority alone has long been discredited.

Even Nikita Khrushchev believed in incentives. He left a memorable quote when he said, "Call it what you will, incentives are what gets people to work harder".

In the US, health care institutions are incentivized by profit. If you lose your client base you go out of business. In Canada, if you lose your client base, in the hospitals at least, you stay in business. Serving patients costs money and makes you poorer.

In the US, the Veterans Administration (VA) Hospitals, military hospitals and some institutions on Indian reservations share this inclination to rationing and causing shortages. They are also on a global budget, where looking after patients is viewed as a cost. There are daily horror stories emanating from American VA hospitals about suffering due to long wait lists and even avoidable deaths. The bench-mark for waiting too long in a VA hospital is two weeks. It seems this goal is seldom met. It is alleged that 40 patients have died at the Phoenix VA Hospital because they waited too long for treatment. The administrators have been suspended. A Congressional hearing with testimony under oath is being scheduled.

Even the great Walter Reed hospital in Washington, DC has suffered from reports of rat and cockroach infested buildings and mediocre care.

The problems with the VA system are no different than the dilemmas we face in the Canadian health care system. The difference is that in the US healthcare problems get talked about and fixed. Not so much in Canada.

My own personal experience with incentives was when I spent four years in New York as a urology trainee. I spent two thirds of my time at a county hospital where all the medical staff were on salary. The other third was spent at a prestigious university hospital, where every physician on staff was on a fee-for-service payment system. The work output per day was at least two or three times more at the university hospital.

Health Maintenance Organizations (HMO) in the US have suffered from patient complaints about denial of care and delays.

The doctors in HMOs purport to specialize in preventive medicine and claim their quality of care is better. But hold on, we need to see some evidence of this. What is not clear is whether the salaried doctor is more successful at it than his fee-for-service colleagues. What is known is many HMOs are against cancer screening. To prevent a death due to cancer is preventive medicine at its best.

Cohen and Solomon,* describe a routine where physicians in HMOs are encouraged to give their first allegiance to the corporate stakeholders before considering the needs of the patient. Corporate

---

*   *Cohen and Solomon, Alternet, April 25, 2000.*

executives have to approve expensive testing and referrals outside the HMO. This raises the specter of patients not wanting to trust their doctors. William J. Mayo said, "The best interest of the patient is the only interest to consider". That may not always be the case with the HMO physicians.

US institutions that work with salaried doctors are striving to bring incentives back into the mold. Most large clinics in the US see switching to a base salary which is adjusted depending on productivity, patient satisfaction surveys and administrative activities as a cure for physician lassitude.

The Mayo Clinic has a salaried system for medical staff. Physicians are kept happy and productive by setting salaries commensurate with the average earnings of others in their peer group across the country. The physicians are incentivized by showering them with academic opportunities, both research and educational. The Mayo system succeeds in attracting physicians whose goal is not to become the most affluent nor enjoy the best life-style, but to aspire to become the greatest and best medical practitioners on the planet. The Mayo Clinic seeks to enable this. That is the best incentive there is.

The bottom line is a salaried system still needs a carrot to flesh out the remuneration package.

Then there are the problems with disincentives in Canadian institutions. What on earth would motivate a physician to treat more patients or do a better job if this results in getting punished for it? This is exactly what happens to the GFT specialists in the Canadian government-managed healthcare system. They have a "soft ceiling". If their gross income exceeds the ceiling they have to return anywhere from 40 to 50 percent to the University and the hospital.

The poor Canadian hospital administrator who is trying to excel and run a well-oiled, efficient institution in Canada will incur a deficit and soon be looking for his next job. Talk about a disincentive! An efficient healthcare institution in Canada, with rapid turn-over of patients, would run out of money by the middle of the summer. It would be rated by the government as a failing institution. The government would likely ask the hospital to close acute care beds until the deficit has been made up.

Chapter 8: Physician Issues

Government Tyranny

THE ABILITY TO PRACTICE MEDICINE WITHOUT POLITICAL INTERference is vital to preserve the sanctity of a good patient/doctor relationship. In the doctor's office there is no place for anything except the patient's welfare and best interests.

The Medical Review Committee of the WRHA monitors the pattern of practice of every physician in the province. They maintain a spread-sheet which documents every public service rendered by every doctor in the province. This practice profile is delivered on an individual basis to every doctor once a year.

With the first offense the deviant doctor is called in for an interview with the Medical Review Committee. If that fails to get the doctor's attention he may face significant financial penalties.

If he sees that he is an outlier he might as well get himself into line – he knows he is heading towards a confrontation. He is unlikely to come away from this unscathed. In the end, he could find himself much poorer unless he modifies his pattern of practice.

The WRHA manhandles physicians who are outside the norm with respect to cancer screening. They do this, not because of public welfare concerns, but solely for financial reasons.

For example, it has been common practice for decades in the United States to perform regular screening colonoscopies to detect early large bowel cancers. Until recently, no controlled scientific study (fourth-level evidence) had ever been conducted to support this practice. The scientific support for screening was based on studies with only historical controls (third-level proof). This evidence sufficed to convince gastroenterology peer groups to recommend screening for colorectal cancers. American insurance companies and American Medicare and Medicaid all covered colorectal cancer screening.

Until about ten years ago, Canadian guidelines stated specialists in this area should not perform regular screening colonoscopies.

A Winnipeg surgeon, a friend of mine, rejected the government guidelines and went with his conscience and peer group recommendations. Because of his conviction, he performed hundreds of screening colonoscopies over many years. The WRHA eventually cracked down on him and took him to court for over-servicing his patients. He lost and was fined $70,000 which he had to pay. (Thomas Jefferson would have called this demand "big government tyranny".)

Ironically, regular screening colonoscopy guidelines have since been adopted in Manitoba, now routine. Sadly, my friend's best-intentioned efforts on behalf of his patients were quashed by government-managed care. He was simply doing the colonoscopy screening a few years too early.

I personally know others who have been bullied by the WRHA for ordering little things, like too many electrocardiograms (he did not own the machine) and too many urine cultures (myself included). It is hard to practice the best medicine in a country that resembles a police state in health care matters.

CP&S and the WRHA

The line separating the jurisdiction of the College of Physicians and Surgeons (CP&S) and the WRHA in managing alleged professional misbehavior and even medical malpractice is getting very blurred.

So far the CP&S has operated without any apparent political interference. They are there to protect the best interests of the public. They have the power to investigate bad behavior and poor medical practice by physicians and levy sanctions if deemed necessary. They also have the authority to suspend a physician's license to practice medicine.

However, I discovered something about Manitoba doctors in September 2015 that surprised me. Having practiced in Manitoba for 38 years I still have physician friends in the province. I ran out of a generic medication for high blood pressure. I needed a prescription for one week to tide me over until I got home. Three close friends in the medical fraternity, former students of mine, refused to offer me a prescription for one week supply, citing fears of CP&S repercussions. I went to the community hospital where the doctor working in the Emergency had known me since he was a medical student 30 years ago. I had been Chief of Surgery in that hospital for over 30 years. He refused to provide me with a prescription also. It may seem petty I would express umbrage over this. However it shows the CP&S has doctors in Manitoba living in a police state. But I think it is worse than that. For all the years I practiced in Manitoba I never charged a doctor or a member of the cloth because of a Hippocratic obligation called "professional courtesy". It was deemed an honor to treat colleagues, especially when they were your former mentor and teacher. There is a loss of mutual respect. It still exists in the US but apparently not so much in Canada. I think socialism breeds disrespect.

In 2004 the WRHA restricted a vascular surgeon's right to perform surgery for reasons that appeared to have little to do with medical standards. The case went to court and the judge restored most of the doctor's surgical privileges. The WRHA was shown to be on a personal vendetta.

In the 1990's there were 20 deaths in the Winnipeg Children's Hospital resulting from botched heart surgeries by an incompetent heart surgeon. Since he was under contract with the hospital and the university the WRHA felt they had the authority to suspend his operating privileges. On the other hand disciplinary actions are supposed to be vested with the licensing body, the CP&S.

Since the health authority has taken on a direct managerial role, for the hospital sector at least, they feel the responsibility is theirs. On the other hand, the heart surgery deaths would clearly fall within CP&S jurisdiction, because of the malpractice. In the end, the CP&S became involved, as it should. The charge of malpractice should never be based on any political grounds.

On the other hand, when there is an administrative or system failure, the government should be held accountable. They have assumed command of hospital governance and should be held totally responsible. In 2014 two patients froze to death in 35 degree below weather when they were sent home from an Emergency Department by themselves by taxi in the wee hours of the night. One was in was in his pajamas and bed-room slippers. This is not an instance of physician malpractice and CP&S should stay out of it. These are catastrophes resulting from systemic derangements in the institution. The fall-out belongs in the political arena. It was the government and its minions that were to blame.

As far as alleged misbehavior of doctors is concerned, the WRHA has medical staff by-laws to govern this. This is acceptable if the scope of the by-laws is limited to things such as completion of medical records and mandatory attendance at scheduled meetings. Malpractice is off limits to political officialdom.

I was physically present when the WRHA medical by-laws were drafted. The bylaws state any disciplinary action by the WRHA with respect to alleged physician infractions can be appealed. However, the appeal process involves essentially the same people as the accusers. This is an invitation to politicians to harass doctors with no proper recourse. There is no independent body to adjudicate the decision except through the courts. In the example of the vascular surgeon cited above, the courts came to his rescue.

Clearly, when politics comes in to play, the dice are loaded in favor of the WRHA. Due process and fairness are suspended. Physician misconduct or incompetence should never be judged by those with a political agenda. The WRHA is a political institution and should consistently recuse itself from any medical professional juristic activity.

Doctor Shortages

In 1991, a government commission comprised of prominent Canadian medical economists put forward the hypothesis there could be enormous savings if there were fewer doctors. They regarded doctors as the gatekeepers of healthcare. They alleged healthcare cost inflation is caused by too many doctors ordering expensive tests and treatments, many of them unnecessary. Gullible provincial government authorities bought into this flawed thinking and summarily reduced medical school enrollment across Canada by 30 per cent.

Five years later, when the smaller class-sizes graduated the country was faced with a perfect storm. There was increased demand because people were living longer and consuming more services and there were fewer providers. A desperate medical manpower ensued. People could not find doctors to care for them.

Soon the shortage in medical manpower reached critical dimensions, especially in rural communities. The only solution was to recruit doctors from third world countries. Sources for doctors were found in countries in Africa and Asia.

To be granted a visa they had to agree to practice in an underserved community for at least two years. Most of them had families. Because of cultural differences many stayed only for as long as they had to and then migrated to larger communities where they could bond with others from the same background. These rural communities are therefore faced with a continuous parade of new doctors every two years.

The mistake has since been recognized and steps taken to increase enrollment in medical school classes. Class size was down to around 50 graduates. This year, in 2015, over 100 doctors graduated.

There is also the problem with home-grown qualified young people denied a chance to become doctors. These highly valued service opportunities are given to foreigners instead of them.

According to a 2011 *Annual Report of the Manitoba College of Physicians and Surgeons,* more than half the doctors (62.4%) based in rural Manitoba originate from Asia or Africa. Fortunately, countries like South Africa, India, Pakistan and others produce an abundance of well-trained doctors, fluent in English or French. A physician shortage is also an issue in urban locations. In Winnipeg (population 742,000), it takes two years to secure a position on a family doctor's patient roster.

Government-managed care (socialism) is to blame for all these problems. None of these problems existed when we had a social insurance plan in the 1960s.

Physician Fee Schedule

Canada's physician fee schedule does not adequately compensate for handling complex medical issues. Some doctors post a sign stating he/she will only deal with a single health concern per appointment. Treating a plethora of problems takes too much time. It is therefore a paradox that patients who require the most care are often the least favored by healthcare providers.

In my Canadian practice, counseling patients with prostate cancer always took at least an hour. I had to explain several treatment options in detail so the patient could make an informed decision. He would have to comprehend the differences between "watchful waiting", radiotherapy, surgery and palliation with hormone treatments. Patients needed to understand potential results and possible complications.

I would always book these cancer discussions at the end of the day so other patients would not be inconvenienced. I would also insist patients bring a close relative or friend to the appointment. A video of the discussion was provided to the patient to take home and review. For all of this, the fee schedule allowed me to charge less than $20, a "repeat office visit". My office overhead was around $100 an hour. I would have fared better financially if I had treated my wife to dinner at a good restaurant instead. It is the fee schedule that is to blame. The physician fee schedule in Canada does not accommodate factors such as time and complexity.

The fee schedule in the US is more complicated, but more flexible. There may be as many as five sub-sections that allow the physician to bill properly. There is a sub-section that recognizes the time spent with counseling. There is a way to bill extra for multiple complaints. A patient with a wrist sprain may need only a ten minute appointment. A patient with diabetes, diabetic neuropathy, heart failure, memory loss and a malignancy cannot be seen in ten minutes. The fee schedule should recognize this.

There is a need to reform the Canadian physician fee schedule. A family doctor seeing patients with multiple chronic illnesses cannot survive in practice unless he finds a way to game the system. This explains why he/she will not report results over the phone, or fill a prescription without being seen. He/she wants to book many quick appointments to offset the service items where money is lost.

Surgeons Opposed to Recruitment

Even though the doctor bills Medicare directly for his services there are still enormous costs that have to be borne by the hospital. A busy surgeon orders countless tests, uses hundreds of dollars' worth of disposable supplies with each operation and is surrounded by a half dozen nurses and technicians. All this has to be paid for by the hospital.

When a new doctor comes along asking for privileges, these can only be granted by taking away from another physician already on staff. There is no provision to add more beds or operating time to accommodate the new appointee. The fixed hospital budget does not make allowance for any extra costs. The new recruit has to win over support for his application from the present-day physicians to have any chance of getting access to the hospital. They have to share scarce resources with the newcomer – a painful dilemma. They are already struggling with an inadequate supply of hospital beds and resources. Patients on long wait lists are hounding the physician. It becomes a heartless and cruel game that plays out. The current medical staff become selfish ganders trying to protect the nest from an intruder.

The biggest losers are the patients out there who are underserviced. They wonder why there are not more doctors. *The Royal College of Physicians and Surgeons* published their 2013 employment study recently. The percentages of new graduates who can't find jobs in Canada are listed below:

Critical Care – 22.7%
Gastroenterology – 33.3%
General Surgery – 28.3%
Hematology – 29.2%
Medical Microbiology – 23.1%
Neurosurgery – 38.1%
Nuclear Medicine – 57.1%
Ophthalmology – 43.3%
Orthopedic Surgery – 25%
Otolaryngology – 29.4%
Radiation Oncology – 51.9%
Urology – 40%
Cardiac Surgery – 100%

It is a very lengthy and detailed scholarly report which confirms the gist of what I have observed on my own. They found that specialists need trainees to help with a heavy load of patients in the hospital but are unwilling to share hospital resources once they have qualified. This results in young graduates not able to find jobs. So what happens to all these young specialists who cannot find jobs? You guessed it. They easily find jobs in the free-market economy in the US. Over there they attract more patients and add value to the institution.

Almost all of the urology residents who trained under me over my 38 years in Winnipeg had to go elsewhere because they could not secure a hospital appointment. I felt sorry for them and tried to help but seldom could.

One of these urologists was especially skilled. He had two years of additional oncology fellowship training in the United States under his belt. He was the son of a local high school teacher and had married a Winnipeg girl. He had roots in Winnipeg. One might argue his home community should give him some entitlement. I was willing to share my hospital privileges with him at no cost to the other urologists. At the time, he was the undisputed best-trained urology cancer specialist in Winnipeg. Surely, he should be able to secure a university appointment and be granted teaching hospital privileges.

For two years, I lobbied relentlessly for a university/hospital appointment for this gifted surgeon. I was determined not to accept "no" for an answer. After striking out at the clinical department level, I wrote a long letter to both the Dean of Medicine and the Chair of the St. Boniface Hospital board, but to no avail. I even wrote a Winnipeg Free Press column expressing my profound disappointment with the recruitment process. After all, three of the four St. Boniface Hospital staff urologists were over 60 years old and due to retire imminently. My endeavors to recruit fresh manpower in urology failed miserably. The candidate in question gave up after two years and moved to the United States. My St. Boniface Hospital headship came under review and I was demoted. I was too much of a trouble-maker.

When I retired in Winnipeg in 2002 I wanted to recruit somebody to replace me. No one "sells" a medical practice in Canada. When a doctor retires he tries to find a replacement for two reasons. One, there is a genuine desire to give continuity of care to the patients. Otherwise, they feel abandoned. Second, there may be 100,000 medical records in storage. The College of Physicians and Surgeons mandates that these records have to be maintained and accessible in case anyone needs them for patient care. A custodian has to be hired for ten years to make the records available in case someone asks for them. It is better therefore to find someone to take over your patient load and in return he/she agrees to look after the patient charts.

I always had the busiest urology practice in the province. I needed a replacement urologist very badly. I found an experienced, qualified urologist in Vancouver to take over my practice. When I approached the hospital board with my proposal, they summarily rejected it. They told me they had heard of my imminent departure through the grapevine and determined my practice cost the hospital about the same amount as the projected deficit that year. They closed the urology service at the community hospital after I left.

Since every other urologist in the city was already far too busy, I have often wondered what happened to all those patients previously under my care.

Thus you have a classic oxymoron: a "glut" of specialists who can't find work and not enough specialists to serve the needs of the people. A government-managed healthcare system (socialized medicine) leads to shortages in a land of plenty.

Precious human resources are simply squandered by government-managed care. Unless something changes, Canada's specialist shortage will never be solved by training more. The solution to manpower shortages can only be found by adopting a free-enterprise system of healthcare.

Walk-in Clinics (Urgent Care)

Walk-in clinics are known as urgent care clinics in the US. They serve a useful purpose in that they reduce the need to go to an Emergency Department. Doctors working in walk-in clinics should get a bonus for working late into the evening. This is when the ER gets the bulk of patients who are not legitimate emergencies.

Family physicians are attracted to a walk-in clinic type of practice because the medical problems are minor and many more patients can be seen in a short period of time. It is a lucrative way to practice medicine.

Walk-in clinics are not a suitable substitute for a primary care doctor. They are unable to offer continuous care to patients with multiple conditions. Conditions such as diabetes, obesity, arthritis, heart failure, kidney disease, mental problems and so on need continuous care, i.e. a family doctor. Walk-in clinic doctors do not do annual physical examinations and preventive medicine. Unfortunately, because of the chronic shortage of primary physicians, a large proportion of the Canadian public cannot find a primary doctor that takes new patients. For them the walk-in clinic or the Emergency Department is all there is.

Reducing the number of doctors has not saved the government any money, as was the original goal. Instead the availability of health care providers has merely shifted from a family practice model to an inadequate, more expensive piecemeal system.

The Hospital-Based Clinics

Before government-insured medical care began in 1968, free clinics were offered at the teaching hospitals. The clinics were staffed by medical students, interns and residents - supervised by specialists from downtown clinics (pro bono). The purpose of these hospital clinics was to offer free medical care to the economically disadvantaged public and offer teaching resources to medical students.

With the introduction of universal medical coverage in Canada, all these previously non-paying patients were given medical cards with billing numbers. All of a sudden, there was an influx of cash. Medical staff debated what to do with this new found source of income. They decided to continue with the hospital-based clinics as before and use the money to hire Geographical Full Time (GFT) physicians. Within 10 years, there were hundreds of GFT doctors employed by the teaching hospitals.

In retrospect, the decision to continue with the hospital-based clinics was a huge mistake. It created two classes of doctors doing similar work but with enormous dissimilarity in compensation and practice opportunities. New non-GFT medical doctors were not welcome in the tertiary hospitals and could not access the enhanced resources in the teaching hospitals. It downgraded the opportunities of physicians working in clinics outside the hospital to the point where independent private multispecialty clinics could not attract the best practitioners. In addition, patients needing tertiary services are obliged to switch to another doctor in the same specialty when tertiary services are needed. The net result is that GFT physicians now have a monopoly on tertiary care.

The government gained complete control over tertiary hospital medical practitioners and recruitment of manpower. All hiring is subject to WRHA approval. This is government management and not a system based on supply and demand. GFT physicians are provided with an office, office staff, instruments and supplies, all at no cost to themselves. They bill Medicare on a fee-for-service basis. Initially they have no overhead and the income is pure profit. There is a set salary ceiling. Once their income exceeds the ceiling they have to return a large percentage of future earnings to the hospital and the university (can be 40 or 50%).

It is very easy to reach your income ceiling if you have no expenses. Once you reach your ceiling you face the prospect of retaining only half of what you earn. Instead of seeing more patients, you might as well go out and play golf or sit on a government advisory committee. This monster replicates itself. The overage (above the ceiling) is used to lure new recruits.

The incumbent outside specialists in 1968 kept their existing hospital appointments and privileges (grandfathered). However, it quickly became impossible for young downtown specialists to gain access to tertiary hospital resources.

The low Manitoba fee schedule eventually created such a differential between US and Canadian physician remuneration that recruitment of GFT physicians became impossible. Steps had to be taken to match GFT incomes with their American professional counterparts. The income ceilings had to be raised. In the private sector, however, the fees did not change as much, tough on private practice physicians and furthering the trend towards a government-managed GFT specialist monopoly.

Since I retired from my Manitoba practice fifteen years ago, not a single private urologist has been recruited in Winnipeg. Retirement and death has led to a 70 percent attrition rate in the independent urology group. The GFT urology group, meanwhile, has doubled.

What this means is that we now see a huge divide between "town and gown". Since GFT doctors have the time and financial support to serve on various government advisory committees and the provincial medical association, there is nobody left to lobby on behalf of the independent physicians. Without a voice and declining numbers, the large private clinics of by-gone days now look seedy and forlorn.

With the virtual collapse of the private medical sector the government is able to assert more and more control over the number of specialists and what they do. Opposition to errant government policy is easily squelched because GFT doctors are so beholden to the government and eager to please. Criticism becomes muted. Government managers are able to move programs from hospital to hospital without objection. Physicians learn to shut up, shape up, or ship out.

Is the loss of entrepreneurial private medicine something that the public will regret? I believe so. The more doctors become civil servants the less personal accountability is shown. When patients wait too long it is never their fault – it is the fault of the system. The doors close at 5 pm and golf is on Wednesday. The phone number is unlisted. If you don't like it, take it to the complaints department. Don't bother me, I just work here. A shortage of manpower supply breeds discourtesy to the consumers.

For example, a friend of mine, a somewhat disorganized middle-aged lady, had to wait nine months for a colonoscopy. Nine months is a long time to remember an appointment. She was fully prepped when she came for the colonoscopy but she erred in coming a day late. There had been no courtesy phone call or other reminder. The gastroenterologist would not accommodate her on the wrong date and seemed to have his nose out of joint. He did not provide her with another booking. Instead, she received a "tray fee" bill for a hundred dollars for a service that was never rendered. That was adding insult to injury!

I can assure you no American physician would ever treat a patient with such callous and cavalier discourtesy and insult. Reminder phone calls are expected. In a competitive world he would be out of business the next day. The Canadian gastroenterologist gets away with such abysmal behavior because he has a near monopoly on colonoscopy. You need competition to keep medical providers diligent and conscientious.

Nurse Practitioners (NP) and Physician's Assistants (PA)

Nurse practitioners and Physician Assistants in the US are a product derived from the military. They are professionals in every sense of the word. Nurse practitioners and physician's assistants have become indispensable in the US. They are seen in most offices, in the operating rooms, on the hospital wards, the dispensary and virtually everywhere else. Most of them are working in a team relationship with physicians but there are also many solo practitioners. Most of them would prefer to work in close liaison with a physician.

Nurse Practitioners (NP) are nurses with extensive additional medical training. They have to have a Master of Science in nursing degree, which takes 2-3 years of extra training. Physician Assistants have exceptional expertise in a defined arena of medical service. Their assigned task may be to give injections to knees or hips, to remove wax from the ear canal endoscopically, to visualize vocal cords, to measure heart ejection fractions with an ultrasound machine, and so on.

The emergence of NPs and PAs in Canada has been impeded by not being able to bill Medicare for their services on a fee-for-service basis. Clinics cannot afford to hire them if there is no way to bill for their services. The only employment opportunities have been hospital jobs. Even here the administration finds it cheaper to use a doctor who can bill Medicare directly and get his pay from a source other than the hospital's global budget. In the US, NPs bill using the same fee schedule doctors do. They can bill Medicare and insurance companies at 85% of what the doctor gets paid.

In Canada, there is an excellent NP service called the Jack Hildes Northern Medical Unit. They provide primary medical care in far remote northern communities. Here the population density is too low to support an on-site physician. These nurses work in relative isolation. However, every conceivable medical resource is made available to them. This includes instant electronic communication with medical supervisors and access to air ambulance services for rapid evacuation when required. The Canadian healthcare system deserves enormous credit for this effective northern health care model.

Within the Mayo Clinic, NPs can diagnose and treat uncomplicated problems, order X-rays, antibiotics, and so on. More difficult medical matters were passed on to me. I performed all procedures such as endoscopies and biopsies. He would also assist me in the operating room. We billed for his/her services. We worked together as a team.

Recently, the Manitoba Minister of Health announced NPs are permitted to order magnetic resonance imaging, laboratory tests, and other medical tests.* This development in Manitoba is a step in the right direction.

However, I am concerned about the cost of the solo NP clinics that are being set up in Manitoba at this time called QuickCare. They do not operate on a fee-for-service model. They work within a fixed budget, a government-managed system.

We are told QuickCare clinics are budgeted at around $800,000 a year. That far surpasses a primary physician's gross receipts on an annual basis. It appears to be a much more expensive primary care model than the traditional fee-for-service physician system.

Employees of QuickCare work a 40 hour week or less, get paid vacations, sick leave benefits and a pension plan. Primary physicians in solo practice get none of these. This raises the point, why become a physician doing primary care when the NP has better working conditions and probably higher take-home pay? What does the MMA, the political lobby for the doctors do? They are politically correct and cowering in the corner as usual.

QuickCare clinics cater to overflow from the ER. They are in direct competition with the Walk-in Clinics, but have a "leg-up" as far as funding is concerned. I would have no problem with them if they operated under the same fee structure as doctors, charging 85% of what a doctor gets. That is the way it is done in the US. This looks like another government-managed system that costs too

---

*   *Winnipeg Free Press, February 20, 2013.*

much. Doctrinaire socialist political motives override common sense once again.

We are short of primary care doctors, both in the cities and in rural areas. We desperately need NP clinics. I strongly support them. There should be no need to bring in vast numbers of doctors from third world countries. In rural areas, these bright young Canadians would blend in with their communities, send their kids to local schools, become civic leaders and make a tremendous contribution. With an appropriate fee schedule, anesthesiologists could hire NPs as primary care-givers and supervise multiple operating rooms at once. Physicians should hire NPs as associates in the office, the operating rooms – literally everywhere.

I favor giving the best economic opportunities in our country to our own native sons and daughters.

Obstetrics and Midwifery

I have family in western Manitoba. Women in advanced stages of pregnancy have to travel a hundred miles or more to get to a place where babies can be delivered. Some don't make it in time and have been delivered in the car on the highway. In the winter the roads are sometimes impassable.

Rural family physicians are not allowed to deliver babies in the local hospital anymore. It is deemed "unsafe" to deliver babies in facilities that are not fully equipped to manage complicated births. There has to be a full complement of trained maternity nurses, an anesthesiologist and pediatric services. There are few towns large enough to afford all these resources.

Even small cities close to Winnipeg, one with a population of 10,000 and the other with 13,000, find it difficult to meet all the conditions on a 24/7 basis. They are open for maternity care only sporadically. Women who arrive in advanced stages of labor sometimes find themselves unexpectedly redirected to a major maternity center an hour away. This has resulted in many close calls.

If it is safe for a midwife to deliver a baby at home, then why is it unsafe for a doctor to deliver babies in a hospital where nurses assist him and light anesthesia can be given by a nurse? Fifty years ago every town with a doctor delivered babies in that manner. It is distressing to see government-managed care introducing restrictions so severe that local maternity services have been regulated out of existence. The pregnant women of rural Manitoba are left with delivery conditions worse than they were fifty years ago.

It must be admitted that childbirth in a small hospital in rural Manitoba might not be as safe as in a big hospital in the city. A balance has to be found between security and expediency. Pregnant women should have a choice, whether to risk a delivery in the local hospital attended by a doctor or midwife or opt for the security of maternity pavilion.

There is an obvious inconsistency in Manitoba Health thinking. If it's OK to perform a delivery in a free-standing Birth Center or at home, why is it not acceptable to be delivered in a country hospital?

To quote Mark Twain, "Necessity is the mother of taking chances". Chasing a delusion of perfect safety can also be dangerous.

In Manitoba, the previous Progressive Conservative (PC) government was just as wacky as the current New Democrat Party (NDP) government. When criticized by the opposition in the legislature about obstetrical services in rural Manitoba, the NDP Health Minister delighted in replying (quite correctly) that most of the rural obstetrical facilities were closed down by the previous PC government.

The popularity of midwifery in North America is on a rapid rise. The patients selected for home delivery are very carefully assessed for risk factors that might lead to complications. There is also great demand for midwifery services in Manitoba and they should be met, providing it costs no more than a physician delivery. If patients pay the extra cost themselves, it should be no one else's business.

Midwifery is an approved service across Canada.[*] In some provinces, like British Columbia, Alberta and Ontario it is funded on a fee-for-service basis. The fees range from $2,500 to $3,500 per pregnancy course. A midwife doing 60 pregnancy courses a year can gross $180,000 a year.

The program in these three provinces is organized along a social insurance system model.

In Manitoba and Saskatchewan the funding structure is a government-managed system. The midwives get paid around $80,000 a year and work a 37.5 to 40 hour week. To maintain continuous coverage throughout the week there have to be at least six midwives to cover each midwifery shift in a clinic. Therein lays the problem. Just to pay the salaries for six midwives would be about $400,000. Costing in the midwife assistant (Doula), the birth kit, secretarial staff, the building and taxes would probably add at least another 50%.

At an average benchmark cost, based on other provinces' $3,000 fee-for-service pregnancy course rate, the number of babies that need to be delivered by these six midwives would be around 160 to 200 a year, just to pay their salaries. To cover the cost of the overhead you would have to add another 80 to 100 deliveries. According to the WRHA annual report in 2012,[**] there were a total of 396 babies delivered by 25 midwives in the WRHA catchment area that

---

[*]   *Canadian Midwifery Consortium, April, 2011.*
[**] *WRHA Annual Report 2012*

year. There were 86 home deliveries, 30 in the newly built birth center, and the remaining 253 at the hospital. The average midwife in Manitoba delivers only 16 babies a year, not much more than one a month. The salary of 25 midwives would total two million dollars. This amounts to $5,000 per pregnancy course.

I have nothing against midwives. I think it is a wonderful service to our pregnant women. I object to the cost. If other provinces can fund midwifery services at a cost close to the fee paid to doctors doing the same work, why does it have to cost twice as much in Manitoba? This is just one more example of how Manitoba taxpayers are getting short-changed by Manitoba's socialist system.

Since two-thirds of the midwife deliveries in the WRHA catchment area are hospital births, the cost per delivery by WRHA midwives costs another $2,500 per delivery. This is in addition to the midwife's base salary. It is therefore much cheaper if the delivery is attended by a physician. The cost of a pregnancy course by a physician in 2003 was $600 in Saskatchewan and $1,200 in Alberta.. When it comes to the cost of a birth in the birth center it reaches an astronomical level. The cost per delivery is $45,000.* Compare this with the facility fee for a birth center in the US. In 2010, the average cost was $2,277.** Manitoba Health says the costs in the Birth Center will come down because the facility is still in a ramping up stage, 32 months after it opened.

Considering WRHA midwives deliver only 16 babies a year, there appears to be an oversupply of midwives. The Minister of Health announced on October 25, 2013, there are no jobs available for midwives in Manitoba.

---

* *Winnipeg Sun, May 3, 2014.*
** *National Partnership for Women and Families, 2014.*

I think the government-managed midwifery service in Manitoba could best be called a government-mangled program. The same could be said about obstetrical services in rural Manitoba.

"The greatest harm can come from the best intentions" – anonymous.

***CIHI Report, Winnipeg Sun, July 16, 2012

Preventive Medicine

I was invited to appear on public television to a panel discussion on preventive medicine with Mr. Garry Doer, who was then a rapidly rising star in left-wing politics. He was the President of the Canadian Union of Public Employees (CUPE). Mr. Doer was a charismatic, unpretentious, impressive, polished future Premier of Manitoba.

His formula for preventive medicine was to provide lavish funding for pre-school programs, teach kids better nutrition and provide properly balanced school lunches, have doctors spend more time on patient education, involve more public health nurses, provide more opportunity for rest and recreation for everyone, raise the minimum wage, and reduce the age of retirement. In other words raise the standard of living.

I responded by saying, "I could not agree more. Countries in the Middle East, like Qatar and The Arab Emirates all have such benefits. Whether Manitoba can afford them is something to ponder. We do not have enough oil wells and gold mines."

"Regretfully," I continued, "there are five major causes of preventable disease and premature death that seem to defy our ingenuity to conquer. These are the five big killers:"

"First, people eat themselves to death. This causes diabetes, enormous cost and premature deaths in large numbers."

"Second, people should stop abusing alcohol and recreational drugs. They are killing themselves at an early age."

"Third, we need to stop people from dying in car crashes." "Prevention here lies with better driver education, better road engineering and policing. There is no role for preventive medicine."

"Fourth, people smoke themselves to death."

"Lastly," I added, "people worry themselves to death. Some commit suicide. The medical profession can play a role with more psych-counselling and medications. But the root cause is economic, lack of proper role models, disintegration of the family unit, loss of a sense of self-worth and purpose in life."

"You see, preventive medicine is only a small part of the solution. Far more important is public education and a return to the spiritual and secular values of our forebears." I continued, "I agree with your contention there should be more patient education by medical practitioners." "The doctors should be able to bill Medicare in units of time spent with the patient, as they do in the States." "Counselling should be recognized in the fee schedule as a highly valued service to the patient."

Mr. Doer drove home the point more preventive medicine could save an enormous amount of money.

I agreed promoting better health is a sound investment, "But only to the extent that we talk about living longer and fitter", I said. "Clearly, vaccinations, adequate exercise, good nutrition and proper doctoring would lead to a healthier population." "The cost of staying healthy must include the cost of detecting illness at an early stage and treating it successfully. There should be more screening tests for various cancers, like prostate cancer, breast cancer, thyroid cancer, lung cancer, bowel cancer, and others." "However, these screening tests are opposed by many, claiming they do more harm than good. I believe the skeptics are mistaken."

"On the other hand", I went on, "It is a sad fact that 50% of the average person's health care expenses occur in the last six months of life. Whether this happens at the age of 55 or 85 it is still the same. The cost of dying is a burden we inherit the day we are born. We cannot change that with preventive medicine." Clearly we are dealing with two things here, the cost of remaining healthy and living longer and the cost of dying."

I sensed we were approaching the end of the show and I planned to finish with my two best zingers.

I said, "I want to berate my colleagues in the medical profession, especially the primary doctors. I can't for the life of me understand why it is impossible to get a complete physical anymore. What is the problem? Does it take too much time? My dog gets a complete physical when I take him to the vet. I can't. How else are you going to detect an early thyroid cancer, a rectal cancer or a prostate cancer? This is called early detection and surely also qualifies as prevention of avoidable mortality."

Looking at Mr. Doer, almost pointing my finger at him, I continued, "Then there is the government and its numerous minions in the "progressive" wing of the NDP. They are adamant in their opposition to screening for cancer on the grounds it is still not established science. There is plenty of proof. What is missing is perfect proof. Meanwhile, thousands of Canadians are dying an avoidable horrible death while the government is obstructing screening for these deadly diseases."

Chapter 9:
Personal Care Homes

PRIOR TO 1969, PERSONAL CARE HOMES IN MANITOBA WERE UNINsured. Clients in personal care homes had to pay the full cost until their assets were completely depleted. Once that point was reached, the province would pick up the tab.

When personal care home coverage came into being in Manitoba in the early 1970s, the personal assets of the home care residents became protected. This was a very good move by the government. The personal care home program is fundamentally sound but there are also some glaring deficiencies. It is mostly a social insurance system but there are unsavory aspects of too much government involvement as well.

Scarcity and rationing is the biggest problem. The wait list for a personal care home bed is far too long, up to two years. Once a client has been "paneled" and judged to be eligible he should be able to enter a personal care home in just a few days. If this is not done, an inequity occurs. The person waiting has entitlement but no services. The person already in the home is getting services, partly at public expense. This is not fair.

Today, personal care home cost is based on each resident's current personal income, spousal included. If one's income is limited to only the Old Age Security Pension (about $600 a month per person), then that constitutes the required monthly fee, the rest subsidized by the Province. If a client has additional income from pensions or any other sources, his contribution to the cost is higher. However, the government caps the personal contribution at approximately $40,000 a year. The average annual cost of a personal care home bed is around $75,000 a year. There is therefore still a substantial government subsidy.

To get a bed in a personal care home you must be assessed by appropriate professionals and prioritized by an admissions panel ("paneled").

Need is not always the basis for getting a bed. The personal care home provides four levels of care. The license might stipulate, because of staffing, there should be a 50/50 ratio of intensive care and ambulatory care offered. Suppose there are two eligible clients, one needing level four care and the other level two. If the bed that becomes available is a level two, the level two will get in and the level four will not. This seems unfair, but is probably unavoidable due to license stipulation. The fact the one with the greater need gets short-changed is obviously inequitable.

The paneling process as it exists today is adequate. Everyone struggling with disabling health issues can be "paneled" and awarded a benefit level based on his current functional health status. A level four client is entitled to the maximum benefit level. A level one client is awarded little or nothing, perhaps just a home-delivered meal per day.

If the need is urgent the client is sent to the first bed available. The client can express a preference and this will eventually be honored. The client is placed on the wait list for the requested institution and transferred later when a bed becomes available. This sounds reasonable. There is therefore much to admire about the personal care home program in Manitoba, particularly the protection of personal assets.

Government involvement in nursing homes should be limited to assessment, allocation of benefits, and regulation/licensing. "Paneling" should be automatic at a certain age, e.g. 75 years. The elderly and handicapped are ill-informed about their entitlement and take full advantage of what is due to them. They manage to cope at home by themselves until they "crash" and then face a long wait list to get into a personal care home. Paneling should also be offered on a case by case basis to the handicapped at any age. Once a benefit level has been designated, clients should get a credit to use as they see fit. They should be enabled to shop for services of their own choosing.

A generic level of care should be adequate care, but could be rather spare as far as amenities are concerned. For instance, accommodations might have to be shared. Private rooms and menu selection might cost extra. The client should be at liberty to pay for upgrades.

Hard-core socialists would object to this. They would see this as an example of a two-tier system. Libertarians, on the other hand, would argue the government has no right to dictate how a person spends his/her own money.

Personal care home proprietors should be allowed to make their own business decisions and be able to add more beds and provide more amenities as they see fit. None of this would need government approval. Personal care homes should compete with each other to attract clients.

The government's only mission is to assure a minimum standard of care and subsidize fees on the basis of need. The government should license the home, make regular inspections, and mandate minimum staffing levels, nutrition standards and safety. The government should monitor and enforce compliance with government-set standards of care. The incidence of bed-sores is a good indicator of the quality of care – this should be public information. Government should also set standards for fall prevention procedures and devices, medication errors, use of restraints, observance of nutrition standards including assisted feeding, dehydration prevention, and so on. Nursing homes should be graded on meeting benchmarks.

There is widespread public demand that personal care homes should be culturally generic. I could not disagree more. Personal care homes should cater to cultural preferences. People in their twilight years are entitled to amenities they are used to. This includes menu choices, staff that can relate to them in their own language, spiritual enhancements and respect for their heritage. The place should be as home-like as possible.

Chapter 10:
The Prescription Pharmacy Plan

MANITOBA'S PRESCRIPTION PHARMACY PLAN WAS FIRST INTROduced in 1971, but continued to evolve until its current incarnation, in place since 1994. This time the Manitoba government got it right.

Pharmacare is a government-owned insurance plan that covers the cost of prescription pharmaceuticals. The retail pharmacies are not owned or managed by the program. Pharmacare is a perfect example of a social insurance plan and not socialized medicine.

There is a formulary that lists approved prescription drugs. If the client wants to use a more expensive version of the same drug he may do so but pay for it him/herself. No law is broken if you insist on buying a non-generic with your own money. A socialized pharmacy plan would prohibit this.

Under Pharmacare, patients with no taxable income have first dollar coverage. There is a sliding scale of deductibles based on the individual's taxable income two years previous. The deductible is 2.8% for taxable incomes up to $15,000. After that amount, the Pharmacare program covers the rest. With higher taxable income, the percentage goes up gradually until a ceiling of $100,000 is reached. From that point on, the deductible remains at 6.36% of taxable income. An individual with a yearly taxable income of $100,000 would have a $6,360 deductible.

Prescription pharmaceutical purchases are tracked electronically by the government. The pharmacy is advised when an individual's deductible has been met. From that point on Pharmacare covers any additional drug costs. You can find out instantly where you are with respect to your deductible by simply contacting Pharmacare customer service.

Other Canadian provinces and territories have different plans for prescription pharmacy coverage. In Alberta residents have to purchase private insurance. Most of the other provinces have a blend of private insurance and public assistance for those unable to pay.

Manitoba appears to have the best plan.

Chapter 11:
Controversial WRHA Decisions

THERE IS ONE REPETITIVE THEME THAT DOMINATES GOVERNMENT –managed discourse in healthcare. That is the desire to consolidate everything. Amalgamation makes it easier to manipulate and exercise complete control. The downside of oligarchy is that it stifles competition, ceativity, personal initiative and resourcefulness.

The WRHA decided it would be more efficient for obstetrical care in Winnipeg to be available in only two hospitals. Because of this change, five hospitals had to terminate their obstetrical programs.

The overcrowding and understaffing at the two remaining hospitals that provide obstetrical services is reaching an alarming level. Delivery suites are occupied and patients have to be transported at the last moment to the other hospital and risk giving birth in transit. This is unacceptable and dangerous. Outside the hospital, in the general community, the problems are even worse. Women in advanced stages of labor are often taken to the nearest hospital, only to be told they do not do obstetrics. The morale among the obstetrical caregivers is at an all-time low.

In addition, one community hospital became a center for orthopedics, but limited primarily to knee and hip replacement surgery. An additional community hospital became a center for ophthalmology.

On the surface, such division of services may appear rational and efficient from the administrative perspective, but it creates enormous logistical problems. Patients often arrive at the hospital with problems in more than one organ system.

For instance, a patient in the orthopedic hospital who has difficulty urinating exemplifies a dilemma. If it proves difficult to insert a urinary tube, the patient has to be loaded into an ambulance, driven to another hospital across town to have this done and then returned. There is no urological service available at the orthopedic hospital. The heart hospital has limited urology coverage. A urinary drainage tube is routinely inserted. Thereupon, the surgery is delayed until they find a urologist, no matter how long it takes. The urology department is concentrated in another hospital. It also means the next patient on the operating room schedule for the day will automatically be canceled because of the long delay.

As an example of the mayhem created by this, here is what happened to Marge and her 90 year old mother in March 2014. Marge's mother lives by herself about one block from the hospital on the southern edge of the city of Winnipeg. At 5 pm, on a weekday, Marge got a phone call from her mother. She had a fall and could not get up because of severe pain in her right leg. Marge and her daughter (a nurse) rushed to the house and it looked like a broken leg. They called for an ambulance. The EMOs agreed it looked broken and told them they will have to take her to a hospital on the northern edge of the city, the only hospital with an orthopedic surgeon on call.

Marge's mother is whisked through some swinging doors of the ER and parked in a hallway, but Marge is not allowed in. The minutes and the hours go ticking by and Marge is pacing the floor in the waiting room, having been told nothing. Finally, after two hours, the security guard is momentarily distracted and Marge sneaks through the doors to be with her mother. Mother is still on the

EMO stretcher and the EMOs are lounging against the wall. When the door to the examining room swings open they can see empty stretchers in there. The EMOs cannot leave until they have handed the patient over to the ER staff.

Finally, after two more hours of waiting, a very angry EMO supervisor arrives, (by now its past midnight), brushes past them in the hallway, closes the door and they can hear angry voices on the other side of the door. The door is soon opened, Marge's mother is admitted and the EMO team leaves.

About two hours later, at 3 am, a very young doctor in a crisp white lab coat arrives and tells them the X-ray shows no fracture. Marge can take her mother home.

Her mother cannot bear weight on her right foot. There is no way she can manage at home. The staff calls for an ambulance to take her home.

Luckily, the ambulance crew is the same two people. They take her straight to the hospital on the southern edge of the city, close to her home. She is immediately processed and examined. An X-ray shows an obvious fracture and she is told she has to go back to the other hospital because they offer no orthopedic services. At this point Marge loses it. Finally, at 5 am, they agree to admit her mother. It has been a very difficult 12 hours since the accident happened.

Since there are no orthopedic services at the hospital they do what they can. She is treated on bed-rest and given a special removable rigid boot. Eventually, she is able to transfer herself to a wheelchair and she is discharged. She spent a whole month in the hospital.

If the hospitals were not government-managed and were operating under an independent administration, government regulators would pounce on mismanagement and insist on improvement. It is unlikely to happen if the government itself is running the show.

The proper role of government should be to regulate. This is severely impeded by the obvious conflict of interest.

Let's all give a great round of applause for the blessings of government-managed healthcare!

Another controversial decision was to have rural hospitals keep their Emergency Department open on a rotational basis with two or three other hospitals within 50 miles of each other.

In Manitoba, when you are driving on the highway and your youngster aspirates a candy or a peanut, and you drive furiously to the next town to get medical assistance, you may be out of luck. Yes, there is a sign on the highway with a big H pointing toward the town. However, there is no one there to help you. It is not their turn to have an open ER. The nearest open ER may be 50 miles down the road. Bad luck!

Chapter 12:
Evidence-Based Medicine

THE TERM EVIDENCE-BASED MEDICINE IS THE POLITICALLY correct name for cook-book medicine. Practitioners of this philosophy eschew anything that smacks of intuition or common sense. If it has not been studied in a properly designed clinical trial it should be disregarded. Some obvious traditional practices like a complete annual physical examination, including cavity exploration, is unproven science and lacks validity. Patients can go for an annual physical and have the complete examination done without the physician ever getting up from behind his desk.

What a government-managed healthcare system is all about is uniformity. It is Orwellian in concept. To paraphrase George Orwell, everything should be equal and the same. To achieve this goal you hire "experts" who draft guidelines, which must be obeyed. Deviation from guidelines is not tolerated and usually results in penalties.

Confidence Levels

Scientists recognize four levels of proof.

The first level of evidence would be anecdotal. There is a lot of it around. An example would be when a friend tells you he feels better and loses weight when eating a cave-man diet. You probably would not want to publish a book based on such flimsy proof. However, it might convince someone to try to live on rodents and rabbits.

The second level of evidence would be if a renowned expert in dietary management recommended a cave-man diet. It could be Dr. Oz on television. He is not a scientist, but an inspiring communicator with a general interest in health. His recommendation is a smidgen more reliable. However, it is still only an opinion based on a review of the relevant lay literature on the subject.

The third level would be research based on a large population of subjects but without concurrent controls. A comparison is made before and after an intervention. These are so-called "historical controls". The trouble is that other unrelated factors might have crept into the picture and influenced the outcome. For example, with PSA early detection research, there might also have been concomitant improvements in treatment. Research based on these kinds if data is usually not accepted for publication in the most vaunted peer-reviewed journals.

The fourth level of evidence would be experiments with concurrent controls. The cases are carefully randomized. There are at least two large populations that are as closely matched as possible. The only variable is the question being studied. The cases may even be switched over half way through the trial (double-blinded) to see if there may be very subtle differences.

Fourth level studies are the only ones accepted for publication in the most highly respected journals.

There is a whole new subspecialty in Medicine, consisting mostly of PHDs who labor in the bowels of the University, evaluating published reports in leading peer-reviewed medical journals. They are not clinicians and never examine a patient. They arrive at sweeping conclusions about efficacy and effectiveness based on what they read.

These non-medical public health scientists devise the algorithms and guidelines that are the basis for modern "evidence-based" medical practice. The biggest drawback to this approach is the best journals only publish articles based on the highest level of proof. Sometimes, the highest level of evidence is not obtainable.

Consider an attempt to show that the Prostate Specific Antigen (PSA) test is efficacious. The study involved 15,000 men in each group over a 15 year period. It was attempted in both Europe and America. Unfortunately, too many men in the control group "chickened-out" and got tested when they shouldn't have. The study cannot be published in a good journal because it is so badly flawed. Therefore, since there are no large successful trials, the public health scientist blithely recommends to the policy maker, "There is no proof PSA testing has any value." He ignores the fact it has been impossible to get the best level of proof. The public health scientist disregards any lesser studies.

When guidelines are being drafted the clinicians working in the field are excluded. It is presumed they are too close to the patients, which downgrades their ability to be objective and impartial. But these are also the people who know what they are talking about.

Too many primary physicians regard these spurious guidelines, drafted by the public health scientists, as gospel. It is claimed these guidelines are promulgated by experts with peerless, untainted objectivity. In government-managed healthcare economies these guidelines are quickly adopted as policy. Doctors who ignore the guideline are subject to penalties. Hence, primary physicians in those countries do not screen for cancer.

In countries with free-market healthcare economies, the guidelines are treated as merely advisory and mostly ignored. If they miss an early sign of cancer they often find themselves getting sued. I know a primary physician in Minneapolis who was successfully sued for millions of dollars for not ordering a screening PSA.

Who knows how many patients could be diagnosed at a curative stage if physicians practiced intuitive, common-sense medicine instead of junk science? But who can blame them when the government harasses them and levies penalties. In a free country the physician would do the test, even when it is not fully established to be effective and figure out what an elevated test means. What harm can it do? Waiting until there are symptoms always means the cancer cannot be cured – it is far too late.

My recommendation is to stay away from doctors who adhere strictly to guidelines and algorithms. Evidence-based medicine can kill you.

Risky Clinical Trials

Many clinical trials are so hazardous to participants in the placebo group they should never be attempted.

A few years ago a clinical trial showed conclusively whooping cough vaccine is efficacious. It was already known cases of whooping cough became rare after a vaccine was introduced. Prior to mass vaccination the disease was rampant. Public health scientists claimed there was still not enough proof because it was only based on third-level research (historical controls). They were adamant a fourth-level study be done.

The fourth-level study with concurrent controls proved beyond question whooping cough vaccine does work. The sad legacy remains now dozens of children in the placebo group risked death or have to go through life with damaged lungs.

Impossible Clinical Trials

Cancer of the prostate is one of the most common causes of cancer-related mortality in men, behind only to lung cancer. Almost 30,000 men die every year in America from prostate cancer. About one man in 36 men will die of prostate cancer.

Given these disturbing statistics, we would hope that everything would be done that can be done to diagnose this disease as early as possible and effect a cure. But nowhere is there more disagreement about the merits of early diagnosis. The reason for all the dissension has nothing to do with a lack of adequate proof; it has to do with a want of perfect proof.

The public health scientists are the arbiters commissioned by government to advise them on healthcare policies. They are revered as clairvoyants, similar to biblical prophets, whose pronouncements are quickly inscribed into laws. However, these visionaries are known to be color-blind. They appreciate only black or white. If the evidence is a bit on the grey shade they still see it as black and will blithely dismiss it as entirely insignificant.

There is abundant third-level proof that PSA early-detection is extremely important, but not much fourth-level data. Since the public health scientist does not accept anything other than fourth-level proof, they still maintain "there is no proof".

Sometimes it is nearly impossible to conduct a good fourth-level study. This is the case with Prostate Specific Antigen (PSA) trials. A good fourth-level trial involves tens of thousands of participants and takes 15 years to complete. The cost of such a trial is 30 Million dollars. The trials tend to fail because the placebo group gets contaminated by participants who get tested outside the trial, rendering the data useless. The subjects become worried about their own prostate health, choosing to preserve their peace of mind over the sanctity of the study. Numerous trials in America and in Europe have been launched but results are still pending.

One Canadian randomized trial,* showed a 62% reduction in prostate cancer deaths within the screened group.

The only other randomized trial on PSA screening published to-date has been by Schroeder, et. al.** The study involved 182,000 men in Europe between the ages of 50 and 74 years. This trial demonstrated a 21% survival advantage to those with regular PSA screening. Those with the longest follow-up (over 10 years), had a survival rate of 38%. "This is consistent with experience in the United States, where death rates from prostate cancer have declined by nearly 40% over the last two decades, although the incidence of the disease has been relatively stable"*** (*Large Urology Group,* May 21, 2012).

An example of third level proof is an Austrian study. One Austrian state (Tyrol) offered free PSA screening, whereas the rest of the country did not. Prostate cancer deaths in Tyrol were 54% lower than in the previous five years, whereas in the rest of Austria it was only 29% lower (Obereigner, et. al.****

In the United States, there is widespread PSA early-detection but such screening is frowned upon in the United Kingdom. A 2011***** study found 91.9 percent of Americans with prostate cancer were still alive five years after diagnosis, compared to just 51.1% of those with prostate cancer in the United Kingdom.

The *United States Preventive Services* Task *Force,* (a subgroup of the National Institutes of Health (NIH)), in May, 2012, is a federally

---

*   *Labrie, et.al., Prostate, 2004*

**   *Schroeder, et. al., New England Journal of Medicine, March, 2012.*

***   *Large Urology Group, May 21, 2012.*

**** *Obereigner, et. al. American Journal of Epidemiology, 2006.*

***** *Lancet Urology Global, 2011.*

funded think-tank comprised entirely of public health scientists (no urologists). They urged against PSA screening for prostate cancer in men.

The response from all urological peer groups has been swift and decisive. Those opposed included the American Urological Association (AUA), Association of Clinical Urologists, Veterans' Health Council and Large Urology Group. The *AUA* described the NIH recommendation against PSA screening as "inappropriate" and "irresponsible" - May 21, 2012 press release.

Furthermore, the AUA concurs with the Large Urology Group there has been a 40% drop in prostate cancer-specific mortality in the United States as a result of PSA early-detection. European studies reveal a 21% drop in prostate cancer mortality since the PSA early-detection era began.

The Canadian Task Force on Preventive Health Care (CTFPHC), a federally funded committee consisting of public health scientists (again, no urologists), similar to the NIH in the U.S., reported in September, 2014 that "there is no evidence PSA screening reduces overall mortality among men of any age". The CTFPHC recommendation ignores the fact in Canada PSA screening and better treatment has resulted in a 45% reduction in deaths due to prostate cancer since 1995. Urology peer groups in Canada, representing doctors that actually treat these cancers, reject the CTFPHC recommendations.

All those thousands of patients out there with non-detectable PSAs after successful treatment 10 or 15 years ago must think all this NIH and CTFPHC palaver is outrageous and absurd. To restrict investigations only to those with symptoms means everyone will always be incurable (diagnosed too late). Without PSA screening the treatment of cancer of the prostate will revert to where it was 30 years ago – palliative care only.

With government-managed healthcare "experts" drafting the guidelines based on NIH and CTFPHC reports, primary providers are forced to follow reckless and dangerous advice promulgated by people with no clinical know-how. Thousands of unnecessary cancer deaths will result.

In a free market healthcare economy like the U.S., government funding agencies like Medicare, Medicaid and the insurance companies tend to side with peer groups that actually treat prostate cancer. They have concluded that it is cheaper to cure cancer than it is to palliate cancer. It is a sensible business decision for them.

Nothing is more expensive and depressing than palliative cancer care. Without early detection with the PSA test palliative care is all there is for prostate cancer patients.

My recommendation is that people should listen to and trust people who know what they are talking about. Listen to recommendations from peer groups in each specialty. They are acknowledged experts. For goodness sake ignore the busybodies and naysayers in the public and the government guidelines.

Primary physicians in Canada need to be reminded the welfare of the patient should be their only consideration. Your government is asking you to skip a test that saves thousands of lives. You will sleep better if you do the right thing and ignore the government guidelines.

To the patient, in Canada at least, the only person you can trust is yourself - your own intuition and common sense. Remember that government-managed healthcare is politicized healthcare. A bureaucrat with a high school diploma is interfacing with your doctor and telling him what to do. Unfortunately, your doctor may not have the back-bone to ignore the government advice.

I have spelled out the area of dissent. To reiterate, the only chance of curing cancer of the prostate is when it is diagnosed early with a routine organ specific physical examination and a screening P.S.A. test. On that point there is absolute certitude.

The objection to screening posed by skeptics is that it might lead to overtreatment. That should never be blamed on a test. If a problem of overtreatment prevails it should be addressed by educating doctors and eradicating those physicians who either can't be taught or won't listen. Every hospital has a standards committee that deals with inferior medical performance.

The treatment options include watchful waiting, various types of radiotherapy, surgery and palliative care. The urologist has the tools to make the right decision.

The two data points that guide the urologist's decision are the cell type (Gleason score) and the PSA level. If the Gleason score is six or less he is dealing with a fairly slow growing tumor. He can project a PSA doubling time of about once every five years. Since the tumor is probably not going to become symptomatic until the PSA reaches about 100 he can afford to watch and wait. However if the Gleason score is greater than 7, the doubling time might be 12 months or even shorter. Depending on the age and general condition of the patient (life expectancy) this could be a killer cancer.

Low grade tumors sometimes morph into more serious cell types. That is why patients have to be watched like a hawk.

Now, why would public health specialists want to ignore all this and recommend no physical examinations and no PSA testing? They seem indifferent to suffering and needless mortality.

I once found myself engaged in a spirited debate at an academic venue with an outspoken critic of PSA early-detection. At the end, I posed the following question to the audience, consisting of several hundred university faculty members. What would they recommend for a 60-year-old patient with a PSA rise from normal to twice normal within two years? Almost the entire audience said they would refer this patient to a urologist for a biopsy, including my opponent in the debate. I emphasized such a consensus shows practically everyone believes in PSA early detection after all.

Other Screening Tests

Because I am a urologist, I choose to focus on the PSA screening controversy. However, similar arguments rage in other areas of medicine. There are disputes over screening for breast cancer, cervical cancer, colorectal cancer, endometrial cancer, liver cancer, lung cancer, ovarian cancer and skin cancer.

There is a wide divergence of opinion about the efficacy of screening for other cancers as well. At one end of the spectrum are the public health scientists that review published reports on screening but do not have any clinical experience in the field whatsoever. They are tasked to comment on things they know absolutely nothing about. On the other side are the acknowledged experts who actually treat patients.

Common ground can be found in screening for breast cancer, cervical cancer, colon and rectal cancer and lung cancer. Public health scientists and organ specific clinical experts cannot agree on the need for screening for endometrial cancer, ovarian cancer, skin cancer and prostate cancer.

Based purely on a review of the literature, public health scientists don't even see merit in doing organ specific physical examinations. We should get government decision makers to heed the advice from experts who actually know what they are talking about.

Relevance of Clinical Guidelines

Clinical guidelines should be drafted by specialty peer groups and not public health scientists. If your health care provider proudly boasts that he/she adheres strictly to evidence-based medicine, you should not walk away - you should run. This could be a doctor practicing cook book medicine. If all physicians practiced this way, PSA early detection would not be offered.

There is a medical practice spectrum, with strict adherence to scientific evidence at one end and witchcraft at the other. It is best to practice somewhere in between, close to the scientific end, but also with experience-based common sense. Under government-managed care, there is no room for discretion. The government determines what the physician does.

As we have seen, the doctor in Canada has reason to fear a painful government crack-down. In this electronic age the government is looking over your shoulder all the time, just like George Orwell predicted. Every doctor in Manitoba gets a detailed print-out of the tests he orders once a year. There is a Medical Review Committee that "educates" you if your performance deviates from the norm. If that does not work they hit you with sanctions. I know because it happened to me.

Canadian PSA government guidelines puts the public back to an era where cancer cannot be cured. Socialized medicine can kill you.

Except in a managed-care setting, like an HMO, American physicians don't need to worry about bureaucratic interference and penalties. Guidelines are discussed with the patient and may or may not be followed. In the end, it is the patient who decides.

Guidelines Protect against Lawsuits

The current Manitoba PSA guideline offers legal protection to doctors in cases where patients requested PSA screening but were denied.

A Manitoba patient of mine was diagnosed with advanced cancer of the prostate at the age of 60. He had requested regular PSA screening from his family doctor for years but was refused because of the government guideline. Now it was too late. The patient tried to sue his physician but failed. The court found that because the doctor was doing the government's bidding and following a mandatory guideline, he could not be held responsible.

When I was practicing in Minnesota, a Minneapolis patient sued his young and inexperienced physician under almost identical circumstances. The doctor argued he had been taught there was insufficient evidence in the literature to justify PSA early-detection. He lost the malpractice suit and learned a very expensive lesson.

Chapter 13: Cook in another City

A BIZARRE WRHA PLAN WAS THE DECISION TO COOK PATIENT meals for five Winnipeg hospitals and three chronic care facilities in Toronto, 1,300 miles (2,200 km) away by road. The food is shipped in a frozen state to a warehouse in Winnipeg, set out on individual patient trays, shipped to the hospitals in refrigerated trucks and then "rethermalized" in the hospital kitchens.

The 39 personal care homes in Winnipeg and the two teaching hospitals were not included in this arrangement.[*] This was likely due to logistics or labor union objections.

The WRHA maintains this unusual system saves money and can better accommodate ethnic food preferences.[**] The WRHA claims only about half the food originates from Toronto. The rest, like fresh vegetables, are obtained from local sources.

It should be easy to find out if this strange way of feeding thousands of patients is both cheaper and more nutritious than the food prepared on-site. Is there any independent study to verify the WRHA claims?

---

[*]   *WinnipegHealthRegion.ca, April, 2013.*
[**]   *Winnipeg Free Press, May 4, 2013.*

The Kingston General Hospital in Ontario has received a research grant to determine whether the cooking, freezing and microwave reheating of food could cause it to lose some of its nutritional value.* Reheating might not be a huge concern in acute hospital settings where patients consume this food for just a short time. However, in a chronic care hospital setting, where clients are domiciled for many months, the loss of nutritional value could be something that should be taken into consideration.

This change in food service was conceived by a PC government in Manitoba. They like to portray themselves as the party bursting with good judgment and common sense. In the general election the NDP rightfully hammered the government relentlessly for being so stupid. They derisively called it "airplane food". This was probably the main reason why the PCs lost the general election to the NDP.

A major change like this in food service costs tens of millions of dollars to implement and also displaces hundreds of kitchen employees. Once a program like this has been established it becomes costly and wasteful to undo it. Dean Acheson once wrote, "Controversial proposals, once accepted, soon become hallowed." The newly elected NDP government lost interest in this issue as soon as it gained control.

The current government's spokespeople are now telling the public that patients in hospitals eating "nuked" dinners find the meals more appetizing than freshly prepared meals.

This food service example shows how a questionable government-managed healthcare narrative can be twisted to sound like a glorious achievement. With enough spin, you can make bologna resemble caviar.

---

* *Diablogue, May 24, 2012.*

According to Tom Brodbeck,[*] the WRHA has 15 public relations personnel working full-time crafting a favorable public perception of this organization. It is quite a propaganda machine!

---

[*] *Tom Brodbeck, Winnipeg Sun, July 12, 2012.*

Chapter 14:
Canadian Life Expectancy

STATISTICS SHOW LIFE EXPECTANCY IN CANADA IS LONGER THAN in the United States. The average individual lifespan in Canada is 81.2 years, compared to 78 years in the United States.[*] Similarly, David Hogberg,[**] states average life expectancy at birth is 79 years in Canada and 76.7 years in the United States.

Canadian media are quick to claim this longevity is due to Canada's universal public healthcare system. It is generally inferred Americans are dying younger because they cannot get health insurance coverage.

There are many possible reasons for the varying life spans of those residing in the two countries. In the United States, there are far more guns, more cars and crashes, higher highway speed limits, more obese people, more wars, cheaper booze, more drugs, etc. Avik Roy[***] asserts when life expectancy rates are adjusted to encompass deaths due to fatal accidents, the United States boasts the world's longest individual life expectancy.

---

[*]   *Conference Board of Canada, Feb. 2012.*
[**]   *David Hogberg, National Policy Analysis, July 2005.*
[***]   *Avik Roy, Forbes, Nov. 11, 2001.*

However, the most likely cause for the life-span differential is poverty. A landmark study by McMaster University[*] showed residents in a wealthy neighborhood in Hamilton, Ontario died at the age of 86.3 on average, whereas residents of a poorer section of the same city died at 65.5 years on average - a 21-year difference. The study revealed a vast difference in birth weight between the two groups. This comprehensive study appears sound due to its large population samples having the same health insurance and the same health care providers (Hamilton Hospital).

The less advantaged segment face many negative influences like poor nutrition, inadequate housing and apparel, limited educational opportunities, alcoholism, drug addiction, lack of motivation, scarce positive role models, as well as widespread despair and suicide.

It is therefore irresponsible to draw sweeping causative conclusions about differences in life expectancy between Canada and the United States without making allowance for other possible explanations.

---

[*] *Hamilton Spectator, Aug. 18, 2010.*

Chapter 15:
A Mandarin Snit

Moving on to the topic of Health Authority impropriety, we had a community hospital board member who donated $600,000 for a new CT scanner. He had seen the need, so he stipulated where he wanted the CT scanner to go.

The CEO of the hospital and the Board Chairman were both intelligent and plucky individuals. The machine was ordered on the premise that it is easier to ask the government for forgiveness than ask for permission.

Under a government-managed healthcare system, strict line-by-line, pivotal, central control is deemed imperative. You are not allowed to order even a single paper clip without first asking permission from the Hospital Authority.

The Health Authority went ballistic when they found out this was done without their blessing - too late to cancel anything though. There was still the need for an operating budget. The money for this could only come from the Health Authority.

Patients from the hospital sometimes needed an extremely urgent CT scan. I remember a patient of mine with a pulmonary embolus who had to be sent to another hospital to have a chest CT scan.

Treatment was delayed by at least four hours because of this. This placed the patient at enormous unnecessary risk. We were incredibly lucky that day - the patient survived. Can you imagine having to transport such a critical patient past a dormant CT scanner with the staff to run it and transfer the patient to another hospital to have the test? All this because some bigwig at the Health Authority had a temper tantrum!

Meanwhile, the CT scanner was being used to investigate patients not insured by Manitoba Health. Professional athletes could be scanned the same day. Patients covered by Workers Compensation could be scanned within a day or so. They were not covered by Manitoba Health.

Trained CT technicians were on site. They were assigned to doing routine radiology. They were forbidden to use their special talents where they could do the most good. They could not do CT scans on patients insured by Manitoba Health.

The hospital was not allowed to use the machine on Manitoba Health patients for over two years. Think about it! Two years with a much needed $600,000 machine we couldn't use. The half-life of such highly technical electronic machines is only about five years and then they become obsolete. What a waste!

We had patients waiting for over six months for a non-urgent CT scans at the time.

Chapter 16: Horror Stories

THE PROPONENTS OF GOVERNMENT-MANAGED HEALTHCARE ARE appalled when horror stories are used to denigrate the system. They claim they are not representative, lack verification, and are nothing more than blatant scandalmongering. However, as long as these stories are truthful they should not be ignored. What happens to a single individual is where the rubber hits the road. Most often large demographic studies do little more than obscure the flaws in the system.

Ella's Story

This is how things went with Ella, a close relative of mine (with her permission).

She went to an urgent care doctor because she thought she had a fish bone caught in her throat. During the examination the doctor thought her neck looked swollen and recommended she be seen by her family doctor.

Three weeks later, the family doctor examined her and ordered an ultrasound of the thyroid. This was done six weeks later and it showed a suspicious mass in her thyroid, about four cm. in diameter.

A referral was made to an Ear Nose and Throat specialist (ENT), which took a month. A biopsy was recommended, which was done six weeks later. By now the mass had grown from four cm. to five cm. By now it was 19 weeks since she first presented with a mass in her neck.

The biopsy showed a fast growing cancer. She did not get this report for another three weeks because the ENT doctor was on his summer vacation.

Referral to a Head and Neck surgeon took only two weeks. The surgery was expedited and done three weeks later. The official pathology report was delayed for another three weeks because of a shortage of hospital transcriptionists.

It took 30 weeks from the original indication of cancer to the time of treatment! The subsequent care was satisfactory.

The apologist for the system bristles when he hears this story. He claims this to be unusual, a professional failure rather than a systemic deficiency. At any time professional judgement should have kicked in and the investigation expedited by picking up the phone and use personal pressure to accelerate things. To chase down a radiologist and beg for an earlier appointment can take half a day. It would be an exceptional doctor who would do this on a regular basis. The system is rigged to invite delays. Is this an atypical story? Absolutely not!

Just for a moment, let's compare this with what happens in the free-enterprise healthcare system in the US.

The urgent care doctor (or PN) would have ordered an ultrasound biopsy of the neck mass and it would have been done the same day or the next.

The referral to a Head and Neck surgeon would occur immediately and the surgery scheduled within a week or so.

There must be thousands of avoidable deaths in Canada because of the snail-pace of medical investigation and treatment.

Reverend Harry Lehotsky

Rev. Harry Lehotsky was a noted social activist and columnist in Winnipeg's inner-city. He was honored with Canada's most prestigious award, the Order of Canada. Rev. Lehotsky maintained a blog. On April 28, 2006, he blogged about his personal challenges with the Canadian health care system.[*] The column also ran in the *Winnipeg Sun*[**] two days later.

"Several months ago, I felt some occasional upper abdominal discomfort. About two weeks ago it was a steady pain that got so severe I couldn't stand for long.

I tried to make an appointment with my family physician and was told I'd likely have to wait months – even after saying I was in pain.

Someone in his office suggested I go to Urgent Care. I stopped by there one day and saw roughly 20 people in the waiting room with one physician on duty. After hearing my wait could be 12 hours, I left.

Finally, on Easter Saturday, the pain was so bad I returned. After six hours the doctor said he wasn't sure what was causing the pain. I would have to be referred for further tests. The preference was to assume it's an ulcer until we knew different. He prescribed some

---

[*]   *Harry Lehotsky, Free Dominion- The Voice of Principled Conservatism, 2006.*
[**] *Harry Lehotsky, The Winnipeg Sun, April, 2006.*

strong antacids. He also told me I would be getting an appointment for a barium X-ray and an appointment with a gastroenterologist.

I was astounded when informed my first appointment with a gastroenterologist would be in November. That's not the scope, that's just the first visit with the doctor!

I got angry when I got a letter saying my barium X-ray wouldn't be until September.

Five months for a general X-ray? Seven months for a consultation to schedule a gastroscope? I started thinking, What if, in five months, I find out it wasn't an ulcer?

Whatever it was would certainly have gotten much worse – even inoperable by that point.

For now, I'll resist paranoia. I'm assuming I'll get better. I don't want to change my schedule, both because there's too much to do and it keeps my mind occupied on positive things.

When the pain is bad, I know others have it worse. If it's just an ulcer, I know people who suffer daily with more serious problems.

Friends and family started finding out about my situation. Responses mirrored my own feelings – everything from shock to disgust that I was paying for medical care not available to me. One by one, they suggested, "Go to the States. You can get in quicker there for the tests."

Part of me wants to stay and fight for what I've paid for here. But the pain and the concern of others override any "point" I want to make with the system.

Yesterday, a pastor friend of mine was visiting from North Dakota. Hearing my plight, he commented, "I know a great gastroenterologist. I'll give him a call." A short while later, I was talking to a doctor in North Dakota. After reviewing my symptoms and the schedule he said he more resources, people wait longer and longer for even basic diagnostic tests that could reduce long-term costs as problems fester during long delays.

Maybe I'll become another poster child for NDP healthcare "improvements". Seven years ago they promised to end hallway medicine in six months.

Not only has that not happened, but now it's worse.

It seems part of this government's strategy on getting people out of hospital hallways is to leave them on the street in pain."

Publication of the column in the *Winnipeg Sun* brought an instant positive response to his dilemma. His case immediately moved up on the waiting list and he underwent the necessary medical investigations in Manitoba.

Unfortunately, Rev. Lehotsky was diagnosed with terminal cancer of the pancreas at the age of 49 in May, 2006 (less than a month after he wrote his column). He died on November 11, 2000.

Brian Sinclair

What happened to Brian Sinclair on September 28, 2008 became a media sensation across Canada. Mr. Sinclair, an aboriginal, diabetic, bilateral lower limb amputee lived in a provincial assisted living abode in Winnipeg's inner city, close to the largest hospital in the province.

According to media reports, Mr. Sinclair was sent by cab to the emergency room with a note from a care-worker to have a blocked

---

* *Canadian Press, June 2, 2013.*

bladder drainage tube changed. He was unable to urinate on his own.

He sat there for 34 hours without getting help. A casual bystander eventually noticed he was deceased and notified the nurse. It is estimated he might have been dead for seven hours. An autopsy revealed he died of a massive blood infection related to his obstructed urinary flow.

The initial statement from the hospital spokesperson was that he was never registered as a patient. The emergency department staff thought he was just a trespassing vagrant, trying to stay warm on a cold winter night. However, this story was subsequently shown to be false.

A video camera recording in the emergency room showed him checking in at the admissions desk. He then wheeled himself to the waiting room to wait his turn. The admission papers were lost and never recovered.

He sat right under the nose of four shifts of security guards for all this time. The camera showed that he was vomiting.

Four years later,* an inquest was convened. It was revealed the hospital held an internal incident review immediately after the event. The findings were kept secret. A "leak" to the media during the inquest disclosed at least four members of the public alerted staff to Mr. Sinclair's distress during the many hours before he died. In addition, several security guards attempted the same. All this emerged as new information. The hospital officials knew about this from the start, but chose not to divulge it to the judicial inquiry.

---

*   *Winnipeg Free Press, March 21, 2012.*

The moral of the story is when the hospital is run by a government agency (the WRHA), and the watchdog also works for the government, a conspiracy to cover-up is altogether much too easy.

Woman Died in ER Waiting Room

According to a blog entry by Jon Gerard, Leader of the Manitoba Liberal party, January 9, 2012,* a Winnipeg woman, Dorothy Madden, age 74, suffered a fatal cardiac arrest in the ER waiting room on September 25, 2003. She presented with typical heart attack symptoms at a Winnipeg teaching hospital emergency room. She was having severe chest pain and was vomiting. Numerous attempts by the daughter, who was with her, to get some action were to no avail. She was still sitting in the waiting room when she died six hours later. There was a public inquiry by the government. Remedial policy changes were recommended. Mr. Gerard's blog entry complains that the inquiry recommendations had not been implemented nine years later.

Not a Good Day

A lady from rural Manitoba wrote a letter to the editor, *Winnipeg Free Press* October 8, 2011.** She said that in September, 2010, she consulted her family doctor because she could no longer deal with her back pain. She needed an appointment for an MRI, first available date February 25, 2011 (6 months since she first complained). She received the MRI result on March 3 and her doctor immediately arranged an appointment with a neurosurgeon. The date was confirmed for August 22 (11 months). She was scheduled for surgery for 11:45 am. October 5 (13 months). At 8:45 that morning, she

---

*   Jon Gerard, Blog, January 9, 2012
** Winnipeg Free Press, Oct. 8, 2011.

received a call from the hospital saying they were canceling her surgery because there were no beds available. She was now scheduled for surgery December 14 (14 months).

Sackville, Nova Scotia

Winnipeg does not have a monopoly on egregious health care problems in Canada.

The *Winnipeg Free Press*, July 30, 2011,* reported the story of a young woman living in Sackville, Nova Scotia with her two children. She weighed 372 pounds. It was determined she needed stomach surgery to help with weight reduction. About 70 weight-loss stomach operations were performed annually in her community.

There were 2,000 people in line ahead of her. In fact, the waiting list for this kind of surgery was over 10 years long! Desperate, the woman proceeded to post her own death notice on the internet.

Eleven-Year Wait List

On Feb 25, 2013, CBC News** reported the story of a Nova Scotia woman who has waited 11 years for surgery to fix a foot deformity (bunions). She can't sleep at night because the pain wakes her up every hour or so. Her surgeon has now left the province and she has to start all over again on another surgeon's wait list.

---

* *Winnipeg Free Press, July 30, 2011.*
** *CBC News, Feb.25, 2013*

Two and a Half Hour Wait for an Ambulance

On October 9, 2012,* a Winnipeg woman injured in a car crash waited two and a half hours for an ambulance to arrive at her location in the Winnipeg. All this time, she was in the care of firefighters who had moved her to a nearby business to wait. By the time the ambulance arrived, her car had been towed away and the building damaged by the crash already boarded up.

The city maintains it is not a shortage of ambulances that causes such a delay. The problem occurs when patients are transferred by ambulance to the emergency department. Sometimes hospital staff is not able to receive the patients for several hours. There can be up to nine ambulances carrying patients lined up by the emergency room door.

ER Frustration

On May 16, 2013,** a woman, age 68, waited six hours in the emergency waiting room at Victoria General Hospital in Winnipeg following a head injury. She went home in frustration and was found dead the next morning. She was never seen by an emergency room doctor.

An Access-To-Information request revealed 23,243 patients went home in 2010/11 from the from the Emergency Departments without seeing a doctor.

---

*   *Global News, Oct. 9, 2012*
** *Winnipeg Sun, May 16, 2013*

Patients Freezing to Death

On February 13, 2014[*] two gentlemen, aged 78 years and 62 years respectively died when they were discharged from the Emergency Department in the middle of the night and sent home by cab without anyone accompanying them. The ambient outdoor temperature was somewhere around minus thirty degrees at the time. One of them was in his pajamas.

The WRHA claims that no one in the hospital did anything wrong. Maybe the cabbies were to blame. A responsible cab driver should wait until the passenger was safely inside the house.

The WRHA maintained that they might not have died of exposure. They both might have died of a heart attack. No doubt their heart stopped when they died. Both were solidly frozen when they were discovered.

Who in his right mind sends an elderly person home by cab by himself at 1:30 in the morning in 30 below zero weather? They evidently didn't even check to see if there was anyone at home to receive them.

Bill's Story:

A brother of mine, a life-long smoker, developed a smoking related cancer on the inside of his cheek in early September. His family doctor sent him to an oral surgeon who did the biopsy in mid-January (took over five months). He could not get an earlier operating time in the hospital. By then it was too late. The healthcare system failed him and he died a horrible death four months later.

This was an avoidable death in my immediate family.

---

*   *Winnipeg Sun, Feb. 13, 2014.*

Kay's Story:

My 75 year old sister was admitted to the Boundary Trails Hospital between Winkler and Morden and was quickly diagnosed with a highly malignant lymphoma. An extremely urgent request for an oncology appointment in Winnipeg resulted in a six week wait for an appointment. By then it was too late.

This was probably an avoidable death.

Barb Snowden

A family friend, now in her 80s, was told she needed a bilateral hip replacement in early 2010. She was booked to have the first side done in 18 months. In considerable pain all the time, she spotted an advertisement promoting no-wait hip surgery at a Sioux Falls, South Dakota clinic. She called the clinic and had her surgery within a few days. When the 18 month wait was over, and since she had not cancelled, she had the second side done in Winnipeg.

Improvements?

Federal money has been injected into the Manitoba healthcare system to reduce wait times in oncology. Studies have shown that access to chemotherapy and radiotherapy have improved. However, the wait times to see the doctor after the first symptom and the time it takes to see the specialist and the investigations remain the same, or are even longer than before. To illustrate the current status of wait times, I would like to share the story of what is currently happening with my distant cousin, Dan.

Dan is 83 years old. At our family reunion on September 26, 2015 in Morden, Manitoba he looked gaunt and complained of losing his energy. He had lost 30 pounds in the past few months. He had lost his appetite, could eat only small portions and had a continuous ache in the pit of his stomach. He was otherwise in excellent health, on no medications and had not seen a doctor for years. He needed to see one now but had no luck getting anyone to give him an appointment. This had gone on all summer.

I used my connections within my network of physician friends to see a general practitioner, get an expedited CT scan and get an appointment with a gastroenterologist. The gastroscopy and biopsy was done on October 19, 2015. This showed a large mass in the stomach and the biopsy was reported, "highly malignant cancer".

It took until December 14 to get an appointment with oncology. Cancer Care Manitoba would not put Dan's calls through to an oncologist and requests for call returns were ignored. The oncologist looked at the data and insisted on another CT scan. The last one had been done two months ago and things might have changed. Duh! Cancer Manitoba assures us that the wait times do not affect outcomes. There are statistics to prove it. Common sense tells me that the "statistics" are nothing more than junk science. Anyway, the second CT scan showed the cancer was much bigger and a chest X-ray showed lung deposits. As this book is going into print on January 9, 2016 Dan is still waiting to start chemotherapy.

I submit that four members of my family have had their chances of cancer survival severely compromised by the lengthy wait times for cancer investigation and treatment in Manitoba. I do not think the Krahn family has been singled out or deliberately victimized by the healthcare system in Manitoba. Every family in Manitoba can relate to these stories. The system is broken and needs to be fixed. There is too much unnecessary suffering and there are too many avoidable deaths.

Chapter 17:
Canadian Medicare Malaise

HAVING PRACTICED IN WINNIPEG FOR 38 YEARS I FEEL ENTITLED to make some observations about the status of healthcare in Manitoba.

To the detriment of the public interest, specialist groups have become much too self-serving and intent on turf-protection. The radiologists are the principal villains in this regard. They protect their fiefdom from intruders as vigorously as any of the most venal craft guilds in Medieval Europe.

Newer technology should be rushed into the hands of caregivers as quickly as possible. For instance, there are cheap, hand-held, ultrasound devices available that can scan for organ enlargement, vessel occlusion, heart enlargement and a host of other things. The technology is easy to learn. The ultrasound machine should augment the stethoscope hanging around the family doctor's neck. He should use it whenever he does a complete physical. It would not detract from the work of the radiologist. Significant findings would have to be confirmed with more sophisticated equipment under his control. The family physician's ability to do an annual physical would be enormously enhanced.

Other professions, like veterinary medicine practitioners and dentistry, make use of new technology as soon as it becomes available. Our primary physicians, on the other hand, remain mired in parochial politics and outdated technology.

In the US, there are businesses offering total body ultrasound scans without physician referral. They advertise on television to scan the major arteries, the heart and the abdomen for $70 and furnish a report to share with the doctor. This should be allowed in Canada. Primary physicians should be doing this – they are missing the boat.

Other specialists are equally guilty of self-interested turf-protection. I was asked by the College of Physicians and Surgeons to visit a young family physician in a town 120 miles from Winnipeg who was doing his own bladder examinations with a scope. It was widely assumed I would stop him from doing this. Instead, I concluded he was competent and knew his boundaries. He was saving patients a 120 mile trip for a 15 minute procedure. My urology colleagues thought I was "nuts" to allow cystoscopies by family physicians.

The role of the primary physician has deteriorated to the point where he does little more than divvy out referrals and write prescriptions. For example, I play bridge with a 75 year old gentleman in Mesa, AZ who lives in Victoria, BC. He claims, in the last five years, his young family doctor has never approached him closer than the other side of the desk during his annual physical. His doctor is credentialed as a board certified recent trainee in primary care. He claims to be practicing modern "evidence-based medicine."

My personal physician in Arizona is a Mayo trained doctor, age 35 yrs. She makes me undress completely once a year and examines me thoroughly. When she does the "internal", I suspect she is looking for a mass in the back of my throat.

In my own urological practice, I diagnosed at least half a dozen unsuspected rectal cancers by just doing a thorough examination.

Last year, the Manitoba medical licensing body sanctioned a family physician for failing to examine a patient with progressive renal failure. He was suffering from renal failure because of an inability to void and had a hugely distended bladder. He missed it completely. The problem would have been obvious if he had merely bothered to ask the patient to lower his trousers. An enlarged bladder would have stood out like a six month pregnancy. As I write this, my telephone rings. A friend is on the phone, calling from Vancouver, BC. A mutual friend of ours has been diagnosed with advanced renal failure. The nephrologist, who was supposed to start him on hemodialysis, examined him and found him to be in chronic urinary retention. He is improving with intermittent self-catheterization. This was an identical botched diagnosis.

The point is this; Canadian family physicians are taught it is a waste of time to examine patients. A good annual physical examination, in their training, consists of merely looking at a few blood tests, checking the immunization record and writing a new set of prescriptions. They are practicing what is called by their family practice peers, "evidence-based medicine." Their strength is not the use of common sense. They follow guidelines and protocols.

Much of family practice as performed today could be done just as well, or better, by a conscientious well-trained Nurse Practitioner (NP). At the Mayo Clinic in Phoenix my wife had several endoscopic examinations of her larynx. You guessed it – they were done by a very competent Physician's Assistant (PA). Likewise, I had a knee joint injection by a PA. Unless family doctors shape up, embrace new technology and start doing proper complete physicals again, they should and will be replaced by a NP.

Family practice residency programs have become an embarrassment. There should be emphasis on thorough physical examinations and new technology. They should be doing procedures including basic endoscopy, minor surgery and normal obstetrics. Lesser complaints should all be handled by NPs and PAs.

Family Practice should be the most varied, challenging and most interesting specialty in medicine. It should attract the best doctors.

In some specialties, the undersupply of physicians has reached a catastrophic dimension. I have mentioned it before, the Canadian Association of Gastroenterology, in 2012, reported there is a 249 day waiting period to see a bowel specialist. If the complaint is bright red rectal bleeding, a cardinal symptom of cancer of the large bowel or rectum, it still takes 143 days. A large percentage of clients with bright red bleeding from the rectum have bowel cancers. Can you imagine waiting for half a year to see a doctor when passing bright red blood from the rectum? This happened to my neighbor across the street at the lake. It took six months for him to get a colonoscopy. By that time he had spinal cord metastases from a colon cancer, became paralyzed from the waist down and died a horrible death. There are likely hundreds of avoidable deaths like this in Canada every year because of delays in diagnosis and treatment.

Chapter 18:
Seeking a Political Solution

Manitoba Provincial Politics

IN 1977, GOVERNMENT-MANAGED HEALTHCARE WAS FIRMLY implanted in Manitoba and elsewhere in Canada. All of the elements of a socialist system were there, at least insofar as the hospitals were concerned. There was line by line government administrative control over purchasing, hiring of staff and the dispensing of care. The leftist government in Manitoba aspired to be in the forefront of establishing centralized government control. Projections into the future included the following:

1. Rural regional districts would be set up, each with its own health authority with strict boundaries and separate budgets. Services to clients who had crossed an RHA border would be billed back to the RHA in which they lived. There was going to be no freedom to choose your care provider. If you did not care for your regional doctor you were out of luck. Crossing the district boundary, except on referral, would be forbidden.

2. There would be community clinics in each district with salaried employees including doctors, district dentistry, personal care homes and government-run pharmacies.

3. Hospitals and personal care homes would also be regionalized and administered by the Regional Health Authority (RHA). Personal care homes would present a generic standard of care and amenities. There would be no freedom of choice. Patients would not be allowed to pay extra to get a single room, menu selection or any other preferred choices. There had to be a single-tier for the poor and the rich. Private payment personal care homes would not be permitted.

4. Routine dental care, including fillings, would be carried out by dental nurses supervised by a qualified dentist. This would also be administered by the regional RHA and incorporated into the salaried mix of the community clinics. There would be no freedom of choice.

5. As far as the medical profession was concerned, in a debate in the legislature as recorded by Hansard, the Minister of Health stated that doctor compensation would be fixed for all practitioners at $35,000 a year. Any physicians who did not like this should pack their bags and leave the province.

In other words, the last vestiges of a free-market health care economy would be completely snuffed out.

I decided to become a politician and see if I could do something to steer the healthcare system back towards a free economy.

The election process starts with getting nominated as a candidate. The candidate is elected at a constituency convention where all members of the party have a vote. Candidates for public office try to sign up as many members for their political party as they can. The cost of a membership is $5.00. I spent six months going from door to door to sign up members for the Progressive Conservative (PC) party. I visited around 10,000 homes and signed up 1,200 new members. Since most of these new members were apt to vote for me, the nomination meeting resulted in a landslide victory for me.

Many homeowners want to get rid of a political canvasser as quickly as possible. One of the constituents urged his dog to attack me and ruined a good pair of trousers and took a gram or two out of my calf muscle. That goes with the territory of being a politician.

Some home owners invite you in for a long discussion. The odds are they want to keep you off the street and limit the damage to their candidate, the opponent.

At one home I met an executive of an automobile insurance company who lost most of his business when the government turned automobile insurance into a government monopoly. He was a frustrated and angry man. I had found my perfect campaign manager.

At another home I came across a middle-aged couple whose parent had been sitting in the hospital for over a year waiting for a nursing home. They were engaged in a raging dispute with the hospital. The hospital wanted to move their mother to a personal care home in the inner city where most of the residents spoke another language and the cuisine was foreign to her. If she didn't move the hospital would start charging her a fee of several hundred dollars a day. I trotted out my prepared spiel on the matter.

I suggested at a certain age, e.g. 75 years, all elderly residents should be "paneled". This would be an automatic assessment of physical status and eligibility for benefits. If they were eligible for services, such as "meals on wheels", help with house-keeping, assisted living or a personal care home, they should be offered a credit to pay for this. The client should use the government approved credits to shop around for assistance in the open market.

The way it was now, the lucky person in the personal care home was getting generous government support and the person struggling at home on the wait list got nothing. Yet, both were eligible for equivalent services. It was not uncommon for an elderly person living alone at home, on the wait list for years for a personal care home, to be found dead after a stroke or a fall. They were entitled to support but never received any. It is a question of equity and fairness.

In the waning years of life, residents should be placed where they fit in best because of religion, culture, language and cuisine.

Furthermore, I told them there should be no quota on accommodation availability. If more beds are needed, private institutions should be allowed to provide them.

The role of government should be limited to assessment of eligibility ("paneling") and standards of care. People who pay for a personal care home entirely on their own should not encounter any obstacles.

Personal Care Homes should be licensed and inspected regularly. The government certification should be posted in a public area near the entrance to the building.

The government subsidy for assisted living and personal care home accommodation should continue to depend on the level of taxable income, which would be obtained from the records of Revenue Canada. This is the present policy in Manitoba and I fully support it.

At another home they wanted to talk about the shortage of doctors. They were new to the province and had not been able to find a family doctor for over two years.

I explained the shortage resulted from a decision to cut medical school enrollment by one third in the early 1970s. The government thought, with scarcer doctors, there would be fewer tests and treatments ordered and money could be saved.

Now that the waiting list for a doctor is over two years, the government is importing them from Africa and Asia in the hundreds. In rural Manitoba, over 60 percent of the doctors are now foreign medical graduates. A doctor from Pakistan, for example, is required to serve for two years in an underserved rural community. Because of cultural differences, he/she usually stays for only two years and then moves to the city where there are congruent cultural amenities.

The country folks are left with a continuous stream of foreign doctors who do not assimilate and become part of the community.

Until now, I had campaigned with my own political handouts, which dealt primarily with healthcare concerns.

As soon as I became an official Progressive Conservative (PC) candidate, I was no longer known as Henry P. Krahn, M.D. The M.D. was stripped from my name. My campaign literature was trashed and I was told by my leader, Mr. Sterling Lyon, never to utter a single word about healthcare system reform again.

My campaign literature was drafted by the PC central office. My campaign manager was replaced and I became a quiet little mouse with no voice. Obviously, polls had shown the healthcare system still enjoyed enormous popularity in the general population and my ideas were far too hot to handle. From the point of view of the big picture the PC central office had gauged it correctly.

I continued to campaign, although there wasn't much fire in my belly or spring in my step. My purpose to engage in politics was to restore a free-market economy in healthcare and that was now out of reach. Instead I found myself talking about bankrupt government owned airplane factories, faulty buses being built by a government company, inedible food produced by a government-run Chinese food factory, about the economics of hydro-electric power dams up north, and where they should build a new bridge across the Red River.

I was essentially a single issue candidate who was commanded by my political party to keep my thoughts to myself. Nothing can be more frustrating and depressing.

There was one bright moment in my otherwise dreary routine. I knocked on the door at one house, ready to make my political pitch, and there stood a pretty young woman with nothing on except a broad smile. She beckoned me to, "Come on in." I told her my daughter should join us; she was campaigning for me on the other side of the street. She said, "Maybe another time then, but you have my vote".

Polls showed the PCs were winning and I still had a good chance in Rossmere. However, on the weekend before the election my opponent made one final delivery to each household. In addition to many other promises, he pledged to continue rent controls for at least four more years.

I lost by 600 votes out of 22,000 cast. Not too bad a showing.

The government-run healthcare system is a sacred cow in Canada, worshipped by the PCs just as much as by the left-leaning parties. Indeed, the PCs, made many things much worse.

Family physicians used to do minor surgery and obstetrics in rural communities. The PC government put a stop to this. Rural family practice was virtually destroyed by the PC administration. There was nothing interesting to do out there anymore. For instance, many rural obstetric facilities were closed by the PC government.

Emergency services in rural hospitals are kept open only a day or two a week. If you show up with a broken bone you are sent 30 miles away to another emergency department that is open.

If you drive through Manitoba on a weekend and your wife suddenly feels dizzy and might be having a stroke, and you see a big sign on the highway with an H don't be fooled. They probably can't help you. The Emergency Department may be closed that weekend.

A cousin of mine, age 92 years, was living in a personal care home in a small town in western Manitoba (population 600). He was unable to void at 2 am and needed to have a tube passed. He was taken to the nearest hospital eight miles away, but none of the four doctors in town was on call. He could not be relieved of his obstructed bladder and severe discomfort and had to be taken to an ER 70 miles away.

There has been a steady progression towards unadulterated socialized medicine for the last 50 years, irrespective of which government was in power. Some of the noxious NDP proposals came to fruition under the PC government.

I felt out of step with the PC party. I was obviously not politically correct enough.

My opponent, Premier Ed. Schreyer, resigned his seat. I could have had the seat in the provincial legislature handed to me on a silver platter. I had no desire to snooze in some back-bench with little influence on healthcare policy. I quickly turned it down.

Organized Medicine

After serving for years as an elected member on the Board of the Manitoba Medical Association, I agreed to run as a Presidential candidate. I was duly elected with a huge majority. I resigned out of frustration before my term as President-elect was completed.

Organized medicine, representing the doctors, is there for show and little else. They do not criticize poor government decisions, even when there is an obvious adverse impact on their members. If midwives get paid more for delivering a baby than a doctor gets, or when there is a money-pit called a Birthing Center, organized medicine fails to fight for the public good, or for the welfare of their own members. Organized medicine is nothing more than a toothless tiger.

Organized medicine purports to negotiate fees for the profession. As a member of the Executive of the Manitoba Medical Association

(MMA), I participated in fee negotiations with the government, sometimes until 2 or 3 o'clock in the morning. We would chat late into the night but finally it came down to the government presenting a pay-package and it was "take it or leave it". Organized medicine has no bargaining power – there are no arrows in its quiver.

In 1980, I was President-elect of the Manitoba Medical Association (MMA). I attended a meeting comprised of all senior officials of Manitoba Health and various hospital representatives. An organization representing midwifes proposed a plan to offer deliveries for the princely sum of $2,500 per delivery course. Physicians at the time were paid $650 per delivery course. Naturally, I objected to the plan.

Did the MMA Executive and the Board support me when I reported back? Far from it! An election had created a board dominated by GFT doctors from Winnipeg who were in bed with the government.

The general public, and even the members of organized medicine are deluded into thinking the Board reflects the majority opinion. Board members sacrifice time and treasure when they serve on a board, but not members of the GFT group. They can serve on volunteer boards without it costing them a cent. The Boards of organized medicine are rigged to favor the government – a quid pro quo. Boards of organized medicine are intent on being politically correct and are subject to government manipulation – subservient to the government.

Doctor Strikes

The much talked about doctor's strike is a farce. First, the entire GFT group is deemed "essential" to keep the hospitals operational. The public cannot be deprived of emergency services. The burden of a strike falls on the private doctors. They are supposed to close their offices, turn patients away, and suffer all the abuse from the disgruntled public and go broke while they are doing this.

A medical practice is a small business. Doctors pay rent and pay salaries. When the doctor strikes he cuts off his income stream but does not reduce his expenses. The government saves money during the strike. All the striker does is to threaten to shoot yourself in the foot if the government refuses to budge.

Besides, a doctor strike is not without great risk to the public. I know of a friend in Northwestern Ontario who suffered a ruptured aneurism in his head during a doctor strike in Northwestern Ontario. The neurosurgeon in town was on strike and he had to be taken to a larger center 250 miles away. Time was of the essence and he never made it.

Another instance of a strike with a bad outcome was a personal experience. There was a dispute between the GFT urologists and the Health Authority over compensation for being on call after hours. It did not directly affect me. The GFT group went on strike and was not taking emergency calls from the hospital at night.

An emergency occurred on the first night of the strike. The GFT urologist could not be located. Fortunately, the problem was resolved by taking the patient to another hospital in the middle of the night. He was a patient of mine and the angry family was in my office the next morning wanting to know what happened. I was not on call that night. I told them the truth – the problem was the GFT group had withdrawn their services. They immediately went to the largest newspaper in town. This became a front page news-item in every newspaper from coast to coast.

I found myself kicked in the groin, not only by the GFT group, but also by the Health Authority itself. There is a culture of trying to cover-up whenever possible. I had no skin in the game and saw no need to obfuscate or prevaricate.

An Alternative to a Strike

If Medicare persists on its present course and doctors are eventually forced out of business by inadequate compensation money will be wasted by people going to the ER. Here it costs much more and the service is piecemeal and fragmented.

In a free society the market would eventually straighten things out. Medicare would make a business decision. Is it worthwhile to drive prices below the cost of production and eventually end up with a system less affordable and much less acceptable, or is it better to pay the doctors a reasonable amount?

Doctors do react under duress by closing their office. We saw this in California where voracious trials lawyers caused Obstetricians to stop delivering babies. Soon the California government put a lid on contingency fees and a ceiling on settlements and normality was restored. Something similar happened in Texas. The shortage of doctors was addressed by making the environment for medical practice more congenial.

The strike weapon is not necessary in a free society. A free market economy has checks and balances. Left alone, without government intrusion, problems in the economy eventually sort themselves out.

There is a big advantage if the single-payer insurance company is a free-standing, independent, non-government corporation. They can respond to fiscal demands at a ten minute board meeting, If it is a government entity, there is ceaseless debate in the legislature and inertia.

The Private Practitioners Association

In 1980, a group of about 200 Manitoba physicians launched a new organization to represent the non-university private practitioners, the Private Practitioners Association. The GFT physicians had organized themselves into a cohesive lobby within the MMA. We needed some balance within the MMA to protect the interests of the independent physicians.

I became the group's first president. We hoped to defend the interests of private practice physicians, negotiate with government over compensation and gain access to better health care resources in the tertiary hospitals. For instance, we saw no reason why patients of highly qualified independent specialists had to change doctors when they needed a higher level of care.

The MMA launched a vigorous attack against us. The MMA wanted to remain the exclusive political voice of the medical profession and the government agreed. The issue was decided in the Court of Queen's Bench in Manitoba favoring the MMA position. The Private Practitioners Association ceased to exist.

We should have acted as a lobby within the MMA and not wasted our time trying to establish a parallel organization to deal directly with the government. Dissenting from within the system is more effective than campaigning from outside the organization. Lesson learned!

The reform I would advocate for the MMA would be to recognize there is a gulf between the GFTs and the private practitioners. There should be proportional representation on the board that reflects this reality.

Representation from each group should be on a per-capita basis. If 10% of the doctors in the Winnipeg constituency are GFT they should be limited to only 10% of the representatives on the board.

Support for Socialized Medicine

I returned to my medical practice poorer but much wiser. The public in my riding seemed to share my concerns about the failures of healthcare. They voted for me in the thousands. The two main political parties in Manitoba were not on the same page with me. To them government-managed healthcare was the way to go.

I learned one or two things in my brief political career. Government-managed healthcare finds generous support in places that surprised me.

The primary physicians by and large support government-managed healthcare. Making a good living is easy for them. There is a shortage of doctors; therefore competition is not a problem. A river of money flows into his bank account without worrying about collections or bad debts.

The physicians fortunate enough to be working as Geographical Full Time (GFT) in the hospitals are even happier. They can start a practice with no overhead. The office and staff, hospital privileges, and vacation time are all guaranteed. There is an income ceiling but it is set pretty high. The doctor pays back "overage" to the university and the hospital which can be as high as 50 per cent of future earnings. If you are giving away half of your money anyway, after a certain point, you might as well sit on some government committee or go out and play golf. You cannot find such a sweet deal anywhere else in the world. But is a disincentive to work in the public interest?

The salaried staff at the hospitals, including the nurses, is as happy as a clam. Nurses' salaries in Canada exceed the salaries paid in the US for the same work. Under a free enterprise system much of the work might move out of the hospitals and into private facilities like Surgical Centers. These might not be unionized.

Chapter 19:
Manitoba Health Mendacity

THE PSA TEST IS AN IMPORTANT STATUS INDICATOR FOR PATIENTS with an established diagnosis of prostate cancer. On this point, at least, there is consensus.

When the PSA test was first introduced in Manitoba it took three months to get the results (early 1980s). Some urologists suspected the reporting of PSA results was purposely delayed by the government to discourage physicians from ordering the test for screening purposes. All other test results were always reported within a day or so.

I had a patient who presented with advanced cancer of the prostate on his first visit. Almost every bone in his body was already loaded with metastases and his initial PSA was very high. He began medical treatment and responded, improving dramatically. However, medical intervention merely puts the cancer deposits to sleep for a short period. If the cancer relapses it can happen very rapidly. All those numerous cancer deposits seem to become active at the same time. Patients literally seem to crash.

I was using the PSA test to monitor this patient's progress. However, because of the time lag between testing and getting the result (three months), it was very difficult for me to stay on top of his status.

When the patient began to feel better he returned to work, which involved hard physical labor. At his three-month follow-up appointment it was not obvious his health had declined. However, he said he was feeling tired and requested a medical letter stating he was unfit to work. His last PSA had arrived only a few days before and it was normal. However, this particular blood work was actually drawn three months earlier. I told the patient I needed his current PSA result before I could furnish the letter he wanted.

When the patient showed up three months after that, I had just then received the test result from three months prior. The PSA test was moderately elevated. The patient had lost weight and was obviously struggling. I had forced him to stay on the job three months longer than was good for him. I felt that I had inadvertently betrayed his trust and felt very badly about it. Eventually, after another three months, the subsequent PSA result came back. It was now about the highest level I had ever seen in my practice.

I was so upset about this situation and my failure to properly monitor this patient's condition that I contacted a popular Winnipeg radio host. He proceeded to interview me on air. I lambasted the system delay when it came to PSA result-reporting. Patients were suffering needlessly.

After the radio show, the laboratory director lodged a complaint against me with the CP&S board for having publicly maligned his reputation. At the hearing, I presented innumerable test results, including my personal PSA report, which I had, ironically, received just that morning. All showed an unacceptable three- month delay. I described the case that had compelled me to go public in the first place.

The licensing board exonerated me, and I left the building. I hoped that maybe I had scored one for the good guys. I do not know what discussion ensued between the board and the laboratory director who was also present at the meeting. However, I was pleased to see PSA results returned within 48 hours from this point on in Manitoba.

There are those who maintain that government-managed health care does not mean that medical treatment is interfered with. Think again!

Chapter 20:
Building a Clinical Oligarchy

LET US LOOK AT WHAT HAS HAPPENED IN UROLOGY IN WINNIPEG since 2002 when I left Manitoba. At that time private urology was under attack by the WRHA, but few people could see it. New recruits to private medicine became impossible. Now, in 2015, there are practically no private urologists left. There are only four or five of them and no one under the age of 50 years. Urological services in Winnipeg are now concentrated in the hands of the GFT group. There is no liaison between the private urologists and the GFT group.

When it gets right down to it, building an oligarchy is the only way government can gain complete control over the physician pool. It took me half a life-time to appreciate this.

Once there is an alpha critter at the top, all the others in the pack become subordinate to him and management becomes easy. This is the European model of healthcare administration. The Herr Professor in Amsterdam or Hamburg has total control over everything that happens within the Department and even in the greater community.

My ideas clashed with this concept. I believe in something that is distinctly American. I believe in professional freedom, vigorous competition and raucous rivalry.

Ultrasound Guided Biopsy Test

In the late 1970s, I attended the regular Annual Meeting of the American Urology Association, an important meeting I seldom missed. I heard a presentation on an ultrasound guided method of doing prostate biopsies.

Until then, a prostate biopsy was always done with a needle, guided to the prostate by a finger in the rectum under general anesthesia. It resulted in very imprecise sampling. Sometimes, the needle entered the bladder, the rectum, a large blood vessel with severe bleeding and even the surgeon's own finger. I call it the hit or miss method. It was a fairly risky and expensive hospital procedure. This method of prostate biopsy involved a recent history and physical, routine blood work, chest X-ray and EKG, admission to the day-unit, use of the operating room and the recovery room. The cost of all this would amount to well over $2,000 per biopsy. Finally, since it is a hospital based procedure there is the usual three to four month wait list.

On the other hand, the ultrasound guided method of prostate biopsy is inexpensive, safe and precise. The needle goes exactly where it should. It can be done in the office at the time of the first visit. The result is available in two days.

I was the first urologist in Canada to do these biopsies. Very soon, I was treating more than half of all the prostate cancer cases in the province.

The technique is easy to learn. I took courses in Philadelphia and at the Mayo Clinic in Rochester, MN. I was soon doing dozens of biopsies a month. In 30 years, I did ultrasound guided prostate biopsies on over 5,000 patients. My positive biopsy rate was around 30 per cent, which means I diagnosed more than 1,500 new cases of cancer of the prostate during my career in Manitoba.

There was opposition to me biopsying prostates under ultrasound guidance, not only from the radiologists, but also from my GFT colleagues. To the radiologists, this was an intrusion on their turf. In the end they could not stop me from doing the biopsies; the government eventually came to my aid. However, they controlled the fee for the ultrasound procedure. I did over 5,000 biopsies without ever getting paid a cent. It was literally a labor of love.

The current average price for an ultrasound guided biopsy in the US, according to the Healthcare Blue Book, is $2,237. In 1990, I had a biopsy myself at the Mayo Clinic and they charged me $1,300. Admittedly, these numbers would include the cost of processing the specimens and the pathological examination. I was paid nothing except $50, which was the fee for a digital guided biopsy done in the hospital. Eventually I started charging patients $50 as a "tray fee" to cover the cost of the needle. It was illegal but I got away with it. I never charged anything for using the ultrasound machine.

I never went into the doctoring business to get rich. However, with these biopsies I was running deeply in the red.

The GFT urologists could not get into the ultrasound guided method of biopsy because the radiologists had more control over imaging in the hospital. Instead of supporting me, they decided to oppose me and played as dirty as they could.

I organized a teaching course on ultrasound guided biopsies and 40 urologists from across Canada were registered. I had arranged for the foremost authority on ultrasound guided prostate biopsies, an expert from Atlanta, Georgia, to teach the class. The private urologists in Winnipeg all attended the meeting. Some of them started doing ultrasound guided prostate biopsies themselves. There was not a single GFT urologist that deigned to attend and the residents were not released. They boycotted the sessions. Worse still, the Head of the University Section of Urology trotted out a small paper, which he presented to a local audience, in which he claimed that the digital method was just as good. There is not a single paper ever published in the urological literature that made such a preposterous assertion.

When his paper came up for discussion, I lost my temper. I pointed out that, in his small series of about two dozen cases, there were no PSA levels documented. The PSA level infers the size of the lesion. If he was biopsying masses of substantial size, perhaps as large as a barn-door, successful biopsies could be expected with almost any method. He should be able to hit these lesions with his eyes closed. In my series of over 1,500 cases by then, the PSA level averaged less than ten units (very small cancers). Most of them were not palpable on examination and could never be diagnosed with the digital method.

The divide between me and my department head drifted farther and farther apart as time went on. We were not on speaking terms.

What I regret the most is that lack of cooperation blocked my efforts to bring ultrasound technology to the forefront as part of a routine urological examination. There is so much to be gained with this technology. I presented a paper at the Canadian Urology Association meeting in Halifax on this subject.

Office ultrasound gives a noninvasive assessment of residual bladder volume after voiding. It also tells you the width of the bladder wall (an indication of obstruction), the presence of defects in the bladder wall ("pockets"), bladder tumors and stones. It gives you the size of the prostate within 10%. (This is important when medical treatment is selected.) It tells you if there are stones and tumors in the prostate. Very experienced urologists can also screen the kidneys for size, cysts, tumors, stones and interior dilation. All this can be done in little more time that it takes to do a physical examination.

Urological ultrasound is such a valuable tool in daily office practice I could not live without it. I regret that this technology in daily office practice died in Winnipeg when I left. I would have loved to pass my experience on to the young urologists in training. However, my immediate superior blocked this.

When I moved to the US I found my ultrasound expertise and office use was the standard of good care, utilized by all of my urological colleagues. It is a great pity that Canadian urologists lag so far behind.

The government-managed healthcare system is to blame. In the U.S. with a free-market health care economy there is motivation to innovate and press forward. The late premier of Manitoba, Mr. Sterling Lyon, used to describe socialist policies as, "the dead hand of government".

Holmium Laser Prostatectomy

In 1995, the introduction of the holmium laser brought a new dimension to surgery for prostate enlargement and obstruction. This marvelous machine was also capable of breaking up stones anywhere in the urinary tract and was useful for ablating bladder tumors. The laser machine came at a cost of around $1,000,000. I hired a urologist to help me with the prostate cancer cases and concentrated on this new technology.

The two companies that manufactured these lasers granted me free use of their machines for six months while I worked out the kinks. When the time came to pay for one of the lasers, I raised $1,000,000 by sending a fund raising letter to my patients. The response was overwhelming. Most patients contributed in amounts of $100 or less. All the money went directly to the hospital foundation. None of it ever passed through my hands. Naturally, there was proper accounting and official tax receipts issued by the hospital foundation.

The laser method of prostatectomy allowed me to send 85% of my prostatectomy patients home within six hours of surgery. The average length of stay with a standard Transurethral Resection of the Prostate (TURP) at that time was four to five days.

I charged the WRHA the same fee as did everyone else using the standard TURP method.

At the time of my retirement in Winnipeg in 2002, I had the most experience with holmium laser enucleation of the prostate in North America (HOLEP). There was only one urologist in the world with more experience with this technique, a urologist in New Zealand. He had pioneered this approach. Over a seven-year period, I used this laser in over 1,200 cases. I was giving courses all over the world, including North America, South America, Europe, Asia and Australia.

The government objected to me raising money via a direct appeal to my patients. Talk about trying to stifle a doctor's personal initiative. They must have responded to pressure from my enemies in the GFT urology group.

They subsequently passed a regulation preventing doctors from doing this kind of money raising. Heck, anyone who has ever been a Mayo Clinic patient is automatically placed on the clinic's fund raising list, until the end of time.

The WRHA never acknowledged the cost-saving advantage of the holmium laser technique.

Chapter 21:
Over-regulation of Technology

SPECIALTY GROUPS HAVE BECOME LIKE THE GUILDS IN MEDIEVAL Europe. The most dictatorial self- interested professional group is the radiologists. However, other specialists are also overzealous turf defenders. It is not in the public's interest for the government to enable these groups to erect unnecessary barriers to efficient medical practice.

Family practice has been victimized the most. Country doctors used to deliver babies, set fractures, do minor surgery, give anesthetics, fluoroscopy and read most of the X-Rays. All of this has been stripped away. It has been "dumbed down" to the point where almost everything they do could be done just as well by nurse practitioners.

I visited a country doctor in 2014 who had taken a sabbatical for a year to serve as a missionary in Africa. When he came back to his town of about 1,500 people he found that a new administration had closed the operating room and he was not allowed to remove moles or any other simple procedures. He was completely frustrated and ready to quit.

Primary care physicians, especially in rural areas, should have much more freedom and flexibility in their practice of medicine. They should be allowed to deliver babies, perform minor surgeries, and do most of their own endoscopic examinations. An ultrasound machine should be parked in the corner of every examining room.

Family practice should be the magnet that attracts the most gifted physicians in the country. There should be new challenges every day; variety and all kinds of interesting projects. All that is needed is get out from under the thumb of the specialists and keep the government bureaucrats at bay.

The doctor should be the central character in the hospital. The others, including the administrator, should be there to serve and facilitate. The idea of having a regional health authority with a lay person in charge is ridiculous. It is like putting a non-commissioned officer in charge of the generals. The "authority" should be the doctor and no one else. The government-managed healthcare system has turned the chain of command on its head. No self- respecting professional worth two cents will ever put up with this.

As far as technology is concerned the template that should be adopted for primary providers might resemble the role of the stethoscope. If that was invented today no family doctor would be given the right to use it. To diagnose anything with a stethoscope requires far more training than is necessary to use an ultrasound machine. Yet, with this simple tool a doctor can make an astute diagnosis in dozens of conditions. He can save hundreds of lives. For more complicated problems the heart and lung specialists are used on a referral basis.

Every annual physical should include an ultrasound examination of the major vessels, the heart and the major abdominal organs. It would take no more than 10 minutes to do this. Ultrasound is non-invasive and easy to learn. What would be the harm in doing this?

Veterinarians would feel terribly handicapped if they were forbidden to use diagnostic ultrasound on small animals. Family physicians are just as smart as veterinarians. The unnecessary restrictions imposed on family practice are the result of government overregulation. Organizations representing specialists are the device the government uses to constrain legitimate family practice resourcefulness. This does not facilitate medical practice in the country. It seriously undermines it.

A similar objection exists to over-regulation between specialists. There is overlap between urology and gynecology in the area of female incontinence. The philosophy should be to ensure competence but otherwise let the best person win.

Turf-wars rage between anesthesiologists and ultrasonographers over placement of intravascular cannulas and intraoperative transesophageal heart imaging. These disputes are tedious and unhelpful.

Chapter 22: National Insolvency with Medicare

My friend Keith Knox wanted to know, "What is going to happen if we, as a nation, continue with the current upward trend in healthcare spending? As more and more of our GDP in Canada are consumed by just one budget item, other important services like education, defense, and infrastructure suffer due to lack of funding."

I replied, "Previous Canadian governments have attempted to address this problem by adopting fixed healthcare spending limits and rationing. It was done with the best of intentions. But, like all other socialist endeavors worldwide, it ended up in a heap of inefficiency and waste. Worse still, the long wait lists contribute to suffering and avoidable mortality."

"The concept of rationing healthcare is both necessary and inevitable. However, it should be restricted to those with the least to lose. For example, if a retired 84 year old needs a heart transplant, he might not be eligible at public expense. On the other hand, if a 44 year old school teacher with a young family needs a heart transplant he should be entitled to it under Medicare."

"At present, wait lists and shortages include people in the most productive time in their lives, the time when they have young children to support. It would be better if we limited rationing to those with one foot in the grave. Expensive treatments should not be offered if life is going to be extended by only a few weeks or months."

"As Medicare money gets tighter and tighter, rationing might be applied more and more frequently, but always targeting those near the end of life."

"Rationing has to be decided on a case by case basis. I remember a 94 year old physician friend, who was denied a hip replacement. He lived to the age of 106 in a wheel chair. When he was denied he was otherwise in perfect health. There have to be exceptions to the rule."

"A decision to deny treatment should be made by a disinterested, objective, deliberative body. Pejoratively, critics would likely call them "death panels." So be it, we would have to live with that." My friend was shocked to hear me mention rationing of treatment near the end of life. He pointed out that Canadian courts might consider this unconstitutional. It might be deemed to be an instance of age discrimination.

I replied. "At some point we have to be practical." "There is no other solution to this painful dilemma of inadequate funds available."

I continued. "The illustrious 19th century Canadian medical guru, Sir William Osler, suggested (in jest) that the rising cost of healthcare could be arrested if everyone was euthanized at the age of 65 years. That would certainly do it!"

"On the other hand, a 74 year old Dick Cheney had a heart transplant. If he pays for it there should be nothing to stop him."

"I wonder, whatever possessed our legislators to think they have the right to prevent people from using their own money to purchase better healthcare for themselves. Thank goodness we have Supreme

Chapter 23:
Investigative Journalism

I HAVE MENTIONED THE DEVASTATING DISCLOSURES BY THE Manitoba Center for Health Policy on blocked acute care beds in hospitals by patients waiting for a nursing home and long wait lists for surgery. The news media only report these deplorable stories once and then drop them. Everything is soon erased from the public memory. What a pity! No good comes from a story unless there is persistent follow-up. Surely there are complications and avoidable deaths associated with the long hospital wait lists and cancellations. It is important these be ferreted out and written about. This is called investigative journalism.

Canadians dwell on all the worthy things with their system (and there are many), but they gloss over the bad things. If you don't focus on the shortcomings there can be no improvements. It appears to me the mainstream media are so beguiled by Canada's healthcare nirvana that looking for faults seems unpatriotic. They assiduously describe what the Canadian public likes to believe – that everything is perfect.

There are obvious Medicare deficiencies but Canadians feel offended when you mention them. That no other industrialized nation has adopted a government-managed healthcare system, except Sweden, has not occurred to them. Moreover, Sweden is abandoning it.

In Canada the Canadian Radio-Television Commission (CRTC), is a Federal agency regulating what is said on the air. Harsh criticism of the government can get your license to broadcast revoked. That is a lot of muscle to worry about if you step out of line. About 20 years ago, when I was living in Winnipeg, two local talk-show hosts were forced off the air because the CRTC did not condone their persistent criticism of the government.

In the US, the first amendment of the constitution is the holy grail of the communications industry. Hence, talk radio is a prominent institution, with both sides of the political spectrum indulging in it. Canadians marvel at what commentators can get away with in their broadcasts.

If the news media seem unwilling to criticize errant policies in healthcare, where could the opposition come from?

Academics in the healthcare system fare very well under government-managed care. They sing praises in support of socialized medicine. These are the "experts" called upon for public commentary. This leaves the impression that most doctors in Canada are ecstatic about government-managed care.

Healthcare institution labor unions have a lock on healthcare employment opportunities. There are no "right to work" laws in Canada. Employees have to belong to the union or at least support it financially, whether they want to or not. Benefits and wages of healthcare employees outstrip similar jobs in the US. The average salary of a registered nurse in Canada is $70,000 to $80,000 (*Living in Canada*), whereas in the US it is $68,000 (*US News and World Report*). Harsh criticism of socialized medicine could not be expected from that quarter.

Whistle-blowers in a government-managed economy cannot expect government protection from reprisal. You can only remain safe if you keep your mouth shut.

Research findings by non-government agencies, like the Fraser Institute, are deemed to be hopelessly biased and cannot be believed. Their findings are dismissed derisively as tainted. The Fraser Institute is funded by private corporations.

The Canadian Institute of Health Information (CIHI) and the university present some valuable research reports. However, their funding is derived, directly or indirectly, from the government. No doubt projects are "cherry-picked" to place the government in the best light. There is an old English proverb that says, "He who pays the piper calls the tune."

So where is any opposition to socialized medicine going to come from? It won't come from the political parties in opposition, the news media, organized medicine and healthcare unions or whistle blowers. Therefore, it can only come from someone far beyond the reach of government.

I hope Arizona is far enough.

Chapter 24:
American Healthcare Systems

Moving to the US

IN 2002, AFTER 38 YEARS IN A BUSY UROLOGICAL PRACTICE IN Manitoba, I got fed up with living under socialized medicine. Frustrated as I was with the University I once loved and the government-managed healthcare system I always hated, I started looking for greener pastures. I was hired by the Mayo Health Care System in Minnesota. Since I had specialist qualifications in the US, the move was uncomplicated and easy.

Practicing in the US under a free enterprise system took me back to the wonderful 1960s in Canada. I could work up my patients in less than a week and schedule the surgery the next day if I wanted to. The internecine wrangling with GFT colleagues who were disrespectful, the fighting with radiologists who were self-serving, the juggling of cases to give them timely care and the lack of any recognition were all behind me. I practiced in the US for another eight glorious years.

Henry P. Krahn

Our Personal HealthCare Experience

My wife and I have Medicare insurance, the same as every American over the age of 65. The hospital component (Part A) is free. The medical component (Part B) costs around $100 a month for each of us. We also carry Mutual of Omaha supplemental insurance costing around $330 a month for the two of us, which covers most of our additional medical expenses. This also provides emergency healthcare coverage in Canada, where we spend our summers.

In April 2008, my wife felt a sudden pain in her left shoulder and could not raise her arm above her waist. She saw her Owatonna-based family physician the next day who ordered an MRI. She got the MRI two days later. It showed a ruptured tendon in her shoulder. A shoulder specialist saw her later that week and recommended a tendon-repair procedure. She consented and five days later was recovering from successful shoulder surgery.

In September 2010, I needed eye surgery for cataracts. I saw an Owatonna ophthalmologist the following week and he booked the first operation two weeks later. In addition, after just four more weeks, he operated on my other eye as well.

In August 2011, I injured my back while doing yard work around our cabin in Manitoba. The pain was so severe my wife had to help me out of bed in the morning. Since I am an American resident, I do not have medical insurance in Canada for elective care, only for emergencies. I made an appointment with a family physician in Grand Forks, North Dakota for the next day. Upon seeing him, he ordered an MRI for noon that same day. A diagnosis was made and medical treatment began. Surprisingly, the MRI also showed an abnormality in my left kidney and a suspicious spot in my bone marrow. I have a past history of a lymphoma, so this finding was troubling to my physician. The physician recommended an ultrasound of the kidneys as well as a bone scan. Both scans took place on the same day two days later. Fortunately, the findings were not serious. The whole investigation took only three days. I was impressed with the friendly and efficient atmosphere at the Grand Forks Clinic. I had never been there as a patient before. After the visit, I filled out a detailed questionnaire to ascertain my satisfaction level. An exit-poll like this is routine in most U.S. healthcare institutions. Americans expect this standard of care as a given.

My Professional Health Care Experience

I began practicing with the Mayo Health Care System in Owatonna, Minnesota in June 2002. Within a week I experienced a feeling of professional freedom and relief. It brought me back to the late 1960s when I was a young urologist in Winnipeg.

Medical equipment at the Mayo Health Care System was state-of-the art. I had the best scopes available, an ultrasound machine for my exclusive use, and a holmium laser at the hospital, a new modern office suite, plenty of qualified support staff, instant diagnostic services and hospital admittance for my patients. I could immediately access renowned medical experts in Rochester, MN. It was wonderful for my patients and equally gratifying to me as their caregiver.

Canadians are misinformed when told medical care in the United States is not available to Americans who cannot afford it. One patient of mine needed a cancerous kidney removed. She told me she had no insurance and could not pay. My staff contacted the clinic administration and within two weeks she had Medicaid and was fully insured. No one was denied treatment due to an inability to pay. No doubt the state would have made efforts to collect from the patient at a later date.

Devastating medical bankruptcies are not uncommon. The Affordable Care Act will fix this if patients cooperate and get enrolled.

Patients were generally satisfied with their overall care, as revealed through hospital and clinic exit polls.

The administration cared about their medical staff and respected them. Better physicians attracted more clients and generated more revenue.

In Canada, under socialized medicine, better doctors attract too many patients. That could create a budget crisis and lead to financial ruin. The hospital has to find a way to see fewer patients to stay solvent.

Electronic Medical Record

Electronic medical records are a thing of beauty. No longer is it necessary to run over to the radiology department to view an X-ray. Patient's records from another site within the network are easily accessed. Patients can view their own medical records.

There is economy in that medical testing does not have to be duplicated at another site. Communications do not require postal or courier delivery.

The main problem is providers spend too much time on their word processors, interfering with time spent with patients. This has been solved by hiring "medical scribes" who sit in on the discussion with the patient and document everything that is said in real time. During the examination the medical scribe lurks behind a curtain while the practitioner dictates the findings, also in real time. At the end of the patient visit, the complete report is ready for an electronic signature and entering. The practitioner is then free to see the next patient.

This is truly a wonderful system.

American Healthcare System Failures

I am a staunch defender of American doctors and hospitals. Nowhere on the planet does the average person get better overall health care than in the US. For everyone, rich or poor, the quality is unsurpassed. The delivery of service is without delay and the supply is plentiful. When it really matters, at a time of greatest need, lack of money is never an impediment. I had patients who were enrolled in Medicaid in just one week. Others go to the ER where treatment cannot be withheld for any reason.

But in the interest of evenhanded reporting, there are some glaring deficiencies in the American healthcare insurance system. There is room for improvement.

Even the highly revered standard Medicare system in the US has serious flaws. It becomes available only at the age of 65. It leaves out the children, who are America's hope for the future and the hard working souls between the ages of 18 to 65 who do all the heavy lifting. They are left to fend for themselves.

The Medicare fund was accumulated through life-long contributions by employers and employees. It is run by the Federal government and is therefore subject to pillage by unscrupulous political marauders. For example, the Obama administration had the gall to raid the Medicare fund, in part, to finance the beginning of Obamacare. Medicare is running a deficit and the fund will soon be depleted. What then?

Medicare is no longer as simple as it was at the beginning. There is a second type of Medicare called Medicare Advantage (Medicare Part C). This is a Health Maintenance Organization (HMO) with more benefits but a highly restricted network. Medicare Advantage is too reminiscent of government-managed care. Some providers will not accept Medicare because the fees are too low. Others cannot accept Medicare Advantage patients because of network restrictions. This looks more like a nascent nightmare than a promising health care utopia.

Unfortunately, the free enterprise healthcare insurance industry in the US does not function, as it should, to keep a lid on costs. The administrative overhead is far too high. It is so high that Congress had to pass a law forcing American healthcare insurance companies to return at least 80% of gross receipts to the people who pay the premiums. The exorbitant executive salaries are obscene. The insurance system wastes too much money on marketing and promotions. All these costs have to be built into the premiums and are money wasted.

As a provider, the excessive variation in deductibles and co-pays make the tendering of claims a nightmare. Too often the provider is negotiating a fee for a complicated procedure with a high-school dropout at the other end of the line. Extra people have to be hired by the provider to help with the paper work. I, therefore, strongly favor a single-payer system.

I find it abhorrent that health care benefits should be tied to employment. If you lose your job, there goes your insurance. If your employer purchases a high-deductible policy with enormous co-pays and a mediocre network of providers, you are stuck with this. The employee has no input into purchasing one of the most important protections for his/her family. If you hate your job but like the insurance, you have no choice except to remain in your crummy job. I do not like the fact that healthcare insurance is seldom portable from one state to another or even from one job to another. Changing jobs often means changing doctors.

The person with Medicare, or has a good healthcare insurance plan, pays the provider a negotiated price. The person without insurance, or those with a Health Savings Plan, is typically charged two or three times as much. That is not fair.

It is now possible to obtain the average price the insurance companies pay. All you have to do is google the *Healthcare Blue Book*. It gives you the fair price of any procedure in your zip code. Armed with this information you can ask the provider to render the service at that price. If he/she declines to sign a waiver you can go to someone else. Parenthetically, this is important for Canadians to remember when they utilize healthcare services in the US. Never pay the asking price. Always remember to negotiate.

Obamacare is not the best answer either. Many consumers want an affordable insurance policy with a higher deductible and co-pay, but this might not qualify under the new system. People are sometimes forced into purchasing more healthcare insurance coverage than they desire. Also, the provider networks can be severely restricted, forcing clients to switch to other hospitals and doctors.

On the plus side, US standard Medicare is single-payer, portable from state to state, universal, comprehensive, and accessible. It should be changed to a non-profit private corporation, made universal for all ages, funded by charging premiums (but subsidize low earners), and get the dreaded politicians from spoiling everything. It would be a good beginning.

Medical Bankruptcies

My bridge partner at Victoria Beach wanted to talk to me about all the medical bankruptcies in the US. I admitted that without healthcare insurance you would be skating on thin ice. "However,"

I continued, "You would not be denied the necessary care. They might put a lien on your house."

"With the Affordable Care Act (Obamacare), every American is insurable. There is no longer a barrier to purchasing insurance even if you have a worrying pre-existing condition. If the premiums are not affordable they are heavily subsidized by the government."

"Of the 41 million people previously uninsured, 16 million now have Obamacare. There are still 13 million undocumented (illegal) immigrants without healthcare insurance. Canada has them also, but not in the same numbers, estimated at 100,000. On second thought, the US has ten times more population. The ratio is not much different. In both countries there is Federal legislation that mandates they be cared for in the Emergency Department whether they can pay or not."

"This leaves about 10 million uninsured in the US who refuse to purchase insurance. Some are young people who think they are unlikely to get sick and are willing to gamble they will not get sick or injured. In 2015, there will be a penalty for those not purchasing healthcare insurance."

"Mind you," I concluded, "I am not a great fan of Obamacare." "There are things about it I don't like. But, maybe we can talk about that some other time when we are not playing bridge."

High Cost of Healthcare Insurance

Bruce Clark's column in the Winnipeg Free Press[*] discusses the high cost of health care insurance in the United States from a consumer's perspective.

---

[*] *Bruce Clark, Winnipeg Free Press, Aug. 24, 2012.*

Clark and his wife are Canadians who have lived in California since 1993, and have enjoyed "top-notch health care". The article says, "When my Canadian friends regale me with their health-care horror stories – waiting for months for pain-relieving arthroscopic surgery; not being able to find a doctor; hospital crowding - I'm almost embarrassed to recall my luxurious experiences. In the span of two weeks, I saw the doctor (an orthopedic specialist), had X-rays, an MRI and a follow-up appointment for a cortisone injection that relieved the problem. If I had needed corrective surgery, it would have been scheduled within 10 days."

Clark currently pays a premium of $16,462 for healthcare insurance for himself and his spouse in California. He bemoans the amount to be so much more than what he would have to pay for Canadian healthcare.

He goes on, "My Canadian accountant tells me a combined income of $120,000 would garner $28,400 of income taxes. My U.S. accountant says federal and state taxes on the same amount will run $20,288." The difference in income tax is around $8,000.

He fails to mention that Canadians pay federal sales tax on goods and services (GST), introduced largely to fund health care. This tax adds 5% to the cost of all commodities except groceries. On an estimated annual cost of expenditures of $50,000 this would amount to around $2,500. All provinces, except Alberta, also introduced a provincial sales tax (PST) to fund health care. In Manitoba the PST is 8%, tacking on another $3,500 to his health care cost.

Thus, in Canada he would pay $8,000 more in income tax, as well as $6,000 in federal and provincial sales tax. Totaling these amounts would add up to about $14,500. With these figures in mind, ($16,462-$14,500), the American health insurance costs only about $2,000 more a year for the two of them than they would pay for healthcare in Canada.

Clark and his wife will become eligible for Medicare at the age of 65, having been employed in California since 1993. After that, they will enjoy healthcare at a fraction of what it would cost them if they lived in Canada. There is no charge for Part A (the hospital portion). Part B (the medical portion) would cost about $4,800 a year for the two of them.

He is so happy with his American health care he finds it "embarrassing" to speak about it to fellow Canadians. On the other hand, he writes, "forking out this kind of dough for insurance is rather disturbing – even if the investment could literally save my life".

Isn't a life worth more than $2,000 a year, or about $150 a month for the two of them?

Chapter 25:
Reforming the American Healthcare System

FIXING THE AMERICAN HEALTHCARE SYSTEM SHOULD NOT BE DIFficult. All that is required is to separate Medicare from the government. It should be a freestanding entity dependent on premiums for support. The only government involvement should be to subsidize the premiums for those with low incomes and to provide oversight and regulation. It could still be called Medicare. As a non-profit private corporation the coverage could be extended to cover healthcare claims from any state or territory in the nation and even pay claims filed from other countries. Competition from other countries would keep American prices low.

It should be compulsory, comprehensive and universal for all ages. Pre-existing conditions should not be taken into account. It should remain a social healthcare insurance plan as it is now. It should be single-payer.

The administration of healthcare is a state responsibility. To make Medicare universal from coast to coast there would have to be an incentive so powerful that every jurisdiction in the land would gladly participate. This carrot should be the Federal subsidization of premiums for lower income Americans.

There are Major problems with the current version of government-run Medicare. Since it is run by the government it is subject to some deplorable political manipulation. For instance, when the Affordable Care Act (Obamacare) was introduced, the Medicare fund was pillaged to support the aegis of the new healthcare plan. It does not provide coverage outside the US borders. This is a problem for travelers going to other countries. Medicare is anticipated to run out of money in just a few more years. Medicare remittances are far too low – often way below the cost of rendering the service. It is not good enough.

Affordability

There are many who maintain that universal Medicare might not be affordable. According to the US Census Bureau, May 14, 2014, the median age of Americans is 36.8 years. Only 12.8% of the American population is over the age of 65 years. The Medicare budget would have to be expanded by an enormous amount to cover the insurance needs of all these additional clients.

Also, according to the US Census Bureau, 84.6% of the American population already has healthcare insurance. All these people pay premiums. The money is therefore already being spent. The difference is cash would be flowing into Medicare and not into the bank accounts of the insurance companies.

We know a single-payer system costs much less to administer. It avoids the need for marketing. As a non-profit the savings could be as high as 20 percent. According to the 2011 Annual Report of the Boards of Trustees of the Federal Hospital Insurance and Federal Supplementary Medical Trust Fund, the cost of Medicare administration is only 1.3%. In Canada, the cost of administration of the single-payer system is also only 1.3%. The December 2008 Congressional Budget Office report, *Key Issues in Analyzing*

Major Health Insurance Proposals, states the cost of administration of private healthcare insurance averages 12%. One has to concede that a multi-payer insurance system does not give you the best bang for the buck.

For the provider, according to Woolhandler, et.al,[*] Canadian health care institutions spend 16.7% of their overhead on administration, while their American counterparts spend 31.0%. Gerald Friedman, *Dollars and Sense*, July 11, 2011, describes how American healthcare providers interface with a myriad of insurance companies with diverse regulations. Canadian institutions, on the other hand, deal with just a single-payer. Single-payer is more cost-effective for providers.

Unfortunately, the advent of universal Medicare for all ages would be catastrophic for the healthcare insurance companies. Hundreds of private insurance companies would be out of business. It would be analogous to seizing private property under the pretext of eminent domain when public interests are deemed more paramount. Is it fair to displace hundreds of thousands of insurance company workers by destroying their workplace? Most would be absorbed by the new version of Medicare. The rest should be adequately compensated and given relocation assistance. Members of the US congress are under enormous pressure from lobbyists working for the insurance companies to prevent any reform from happening.

Current healthcare insurance in America, provided by companies as a benefit, binds workers too close to the employer. It was an imprudent device in the 1940s, when labor was scarce, for companies to use healthcare insurance to lure people to work for them. It discourages employees from leaving the company with its healthcare benefits and setting up new small businesses. It is high time this was changed.

---

[*]   *Woolhandler, et.al., New England Journal of Medicine, Aug. 21, 2003.*

One obvious advantage to creating a universal Medicare system would be the removal of the entrenched legal obligation for employers to provide healthcare insurance to their workforce. A healthcare policy is negotiated by companies as cheaply as possible on the rationale of reducing their share of the cost. Higher deductibles, reduced range of services and lesser quality network providers can all decrease the employer's share of the premiums. Employees have no control over this and can end up with higher co-pays, higher deductibles and inferior healthcare coverage. They are stripped of control over one of the most important issues in their daily life.

Financing Universal Medicare

The premiums for Medicare should be based on estimations, furnished by qualified actuaries, of what is needed to fully fund Medicare. If the average cost of Medicare is, say $15,000 a year for a family of four, the maximum premium would have to be set at that level. Those without any taxable income would get a $15,000 annual government subsidy. Those at the threshold level would get no subsidy and pay the full premium themselves. Where the maximum premium kicks in on the income scale would be a political decision by the government. A higher threshold would require government premium subsidization for more people. I would expect it might be around $100,000 taxable income. In between would be a downward sliding scale of subsidies. The money for the subsidy could be raised by levying a national sales tax.

There should be a deductible for everyone. For those without taxable income it should just be a nominal amount. The $147 deductible for Part B with the current Medicare system sounds about right. For those with taxable income the deductible might be set at 5%. Therefore, a family of four with taxable income of $100,000 would have a deductible of $5,000.

The difference between extra-billing and co-pay is extra-billing is discretionary. I prefer to go with extra-billing. Some providers might never extra-bill. Also, there should be a ceiling to extra-billing. Once legitimate healthcare expenses exceed the taxable income level extra-billing should be disallowed. Medicare would notify the client the extra-billing does not need to be paid. Medicare would interface with the IRS to get the taxable income level.

There are some American communities (e.g. Tucson, Arizona) where few providers will accept the current Medicare payment as full payment. They claim the reimbursement levels are too low. Their operating expenses are not met and they obviously cannot survive when operating at a loss.

Medicare needs to continuously make timely adjustments to the fee schedule. The decision to enhance compensation should not be difficult. The under-serviced patients, denied care, inevitably end up in the hospital emergency department where refusal of service is illegal but very costly. Once this becomes more expensive than correcting legitimate pecuniary grievances, fees and premiums need to be raised.

A government agency like the current Medicare system finds it difficult to do this because it is politicized and not operating on a conventional business basis. Any change is subject to an endless debate and approval process in congress. A free-standing independent private corporation can make a commercial decision at a single board meeting.

On the other hand, providers have been known to form a pact or cartel so they can lever Medicare into paying undeserved higher charges. The free-enterprise system cannot control prices when there is a monopoly. Government regulation should step in and deal with this.

In New York state only government-approved less-costly clinics are allowed to treat Medicaid patients. Other states are following New York's lead. This is a return to the discredited network system. This policy leads to the reviled two-tier system many find so objectionable. Americans need to wake up and halt this movement right now.

Elite HealthCare Providers

There is always going to be a need for institutions with higher than standard levels of care – elite healthcare providers. These institutions make an extraordinary commitment to excellence. They are in the forefront of medical education and research. They attract physicians with an international reputation and draw clients from far and wide. An elite provider gets all the extremely complicated, uncommon and baffling cases. Special expertise is needed and has to be paid for. To achieve elite status should not be easy.

Medicare should pay a reasonable extra fee for clients needing superior care. The additional fees charged by elite healthcare providers should be paid by Medicare with no deductible or co-pay, but only if there is a physician referral and pre-approval. Since clients not referred by Medicare are entitled only to a generic level of care, any charges above the Medicare rate would be on their own dime.

I submit this is not two-tier medicine. Referral to an elite provider is not unusual in Canada – a bastion of single tier healthcare. When local physicians request it, Canadian patients are often referred to an elite provider at tax-payer expense.

Malpractice Reform

Healthcare law suits cost an inordinate amount of money. Not only are the judgments astronomical and obscene, the efforts by providers to protect themselves from law-suits leads to over-investigation. This squanders huge amounts of money. Tort reform is urgently needed.

According to Jena, et. al.[*] 100 percent of doctors practicing in a high risk specialty should expect to be sued at least once during their career.

Canadians seem to know how to deal with this. They do this by settling quickly and as cheaply as possible when the case is indefensible. If the suit is defensible it has to be fought with no holds barred. Trial lawyers depend on winning because they operate under a contingency basis. They will not want to waste their time if they sense they might lose.

Other HealthCare Reform Suggestions

There should be a major effort made to recycle "disposables" in the hospitals. For instance, a laser fiber may be 20 feet in length. Only one cm. or so has been burned off during a procedure. Yet, because it is labelled "single use", it all has to be discarded. With proper cleaning and sterilization it could be used for 100 cases or more. This happens with every instrument that is used in modern endoscopic surgery. The waste of perfectly good equipment amounts to hundreds, or even thousands of dollars for every biopsy and every endoscopic surgical procedure. It is mind-boggling how much money is wasted every day.

In the 2012 American presidential election, the Republican nominee, Mitt Romney, proposed a voucher system allowing senior citizens to purchase private insurance in lieu of Medicare enrollment. This plan would inevitably increase providers' costs, for they would now have to bear the cost of dealing with multiple payers. Romney's proposal would lead to cherry-picking by the private insurance companies.

---

[*] *Jena, et. al., New England Journal of Medicine, vol.. 365, 2011*

The high-risk patients would all end up with Medicare. This is an idea that does not deserve further consideration.

Another healthcare reform suggestion was made by the George W. Bush administration. They recommended Health Savings Accounts (HSA), where tax-payers could set up a personal account with pre-tax dollars to draw on to pay for healthcare costs in the future. These would function exactly like a 401K savings plan for retirement. You cannot save enough money this way. What do you do when you run out of money and don't have Medicare? This is not a good idea.

Americans should not vote for a political party that wants to dispense with a single-payer insurance system. The cost of administration for both the insurance supplier and the healthcare provider should be kept affordable.

The Affordable Care Act (Obamacare)

There are three big advantages to Obamacare. First, the pre-existing condition exclusion clause is no longer an issue under the plan. Second, everyone is encouraged to be insured. Third, there are subsidies for those who cannot afford the premiums. However, the purchase of insurance is not mandatory. The result is that a significant number of people still remain uninsured. Surely, they have only themselves to blame when huge medical bills create financial insolvency.

At a book signing in Phoenix in early 2014, I met a 60 year old gentleman from Alberta, Canada who was an immigrant to the US in December, 2013. He had an extremely aggressive bone marrow malignancy and had two stem cell transplants in Canada. He had relapsed again and was denied a third stem cell transplant in Canada because of rationing. At the beginning of January, 2014, he purchased healthcare insurance under the Affordable Care Act with no questions asked.

When I saw him in February, he was already recovering from another stem cell transplant (cost around $350,000), and felt hale and hearty again. Moving to the US gave him a new lease on life, thanks to Obamacare.

There are those who object to an "individual mandate", which would force everyone to sign up for and pay for healthcare insurance. They claim individual freedom is encroached upon. However, when push comes to shove, all these freedom loving spongers get excellent care at public expense. The rest of Americans end up having to pay for this.

Despite these attributes, not all is well with Obamacare. Any plan 1,900 pages long seems much too complicated. (In contrast, the Canada Health Act is only 13 pages long.) When compared to other nations' healthcare systems, Obamacare wins the "convolution" prize. During the Congress debate on the plan, Speaker of the House, Nancy Pelosi, advised legislators to pass the motion and struggle to understand it later.

Albert Einstein said, "Make everything as simple as possible, but not simpler". American healthcare planners should have heeded Mr. Einstein's sage advice.

Under Obamacare many Americans have seen their deductible and insurance premiums skyrocket. Their employers are at fault. Some are negotiating high deductibles with insurance companies to reduce their portion of the premium. Others have found it necessary to change insurance companies because Obamacare deems the coverage too chintzy and not acceptable. Changing insurance companies may result in having a different network of providers. This forces employees to change doctors.

If current trends go on and healthcare costs continue to soar, there will be no money left for other necessities in America. These could be essential services such as education, defense, public protection, research/development and public infrastructure.

It sounds tempting to some to restrain spiraling costs by imposing a Canadian-style government autocracy to control healthcare cost. That would be a disastrous development. Who wants rationing, scarcity, long wait lists and avoidable deaths? Fortunately, the current Canadian healthcare system would never be tolerated in America. The right to pay for healthcare with your own money is protected by the Tenth Amendment of the American Bill of Rights.

American Healthcare System Inflation

This is the final and most important observation I have to make in this chapter. There is a fix to the ever-rising cost of healthcare in America.

American social healthcare insurance should cover clients on a world-wide basis. Hospitals in India and elsewhere have American trained physicians doing excellent work at a fraction of what it costs in the US. They do not have to deal with ridiculous demands by regulators, by outrageous labor union pressures and unconscionable trial lawyers. All this contributes to the high cost of healthcare in America.

Canadians believe their healthcare system cost is lower than it is in the US. If so, Canadian providers could provide an exceptional choice for budget-minded American clients.

If American healthcare insurance was portable on a global basis and subject to competition beyond the US borders, the high charges by American providers would plummet like a meteor.

Discussion

At the previously mentioned book signing in Phoenix I was asked some questions from the floor about American Medicare.

The first wanted to know if the advent of Obamacare has affected the number of uninsured in America. I replied, "President Obama claims 16 Million of the previously 41 Million uninsured are now covered. Of the 25 Million still uninsured there are about 13 Million undocumented aliens who are not eligible to be insured. The remaining 12 Million want to be self-insured or simply refuse to be insured for various reasons."

"There are also uninsured people living in Canada. There are an estimated 100,000 illegal aliens living in Canada without healthcare insurance."

Another wanted to know if I had much personal experience with Medicare in the US. I told them, "I had an accident where I fracture-dislocated my right shoulder. I needed a shoulder replacement."

"I have US Medicare. Part A (hospital), which has a deductible of $1,260. Part B (medical) has a small deductible of $147. There is 80% co-pay for Part B. I have a supplementary insurance policy costing around $3,000 a year. However, this supplementary policy also covers me for emergencies in Canada, where I spend three months a year. US Medicare does not pay out of country providers."

"My bill for fixing my shoulder came to $44,000. I paid $2,000 out of pocket. I think this is a reasonable amount."

"The wait period for the surgery was about three weeks. I could have had it done quicker by others but I picked the best shoulder surgeon in Arizona."

Many questions were asked about the high deductible that I lauded in *Damaged Care,* my first book. I believe in deductibles because they cause people to pause and shop for a better deal. For instance, why pay $2,200 for an MRI at one facility when a competitor across the street does it for $950? Competition keeps prices down.

The discussion on global healthcare coverage got completely out of hand. This is a real hot potato. The meeting degenerated into abusive language and angry exchanges between members in the audience. Some argued the fate of American healthcare might be the same as happened to the garment industry, e.g. Bangla Dash sweatshops. Third world countries with lower standards might become a favorite destination for healthcare. There are those who view this as a threat to high American standards that can be trusted. Others saw this as an erosion of American employment opportunities.

There can be no doubt the cost of healthcare in the US would be affected in a downward direction.

Most people would prefer to stay in the US for their healthcare. However, some might be tempted to get things done cheaper elsewhere.

The point remains the privatization of Medicare takes the program to the status of regular insurance. For example, with your regular automobile insurance you do not worry when you cross the border into Canada. Your insurance remains perfectly valid. So it should also be with healthcare insurance. The current Medicare offers coverage only in America.

In Colorado, a single payer system will be on the ballot in November. To me this looks precisely like the kind of healthcare system that I would endorse - with one major proviso. I do not like to see it associated with employment status. Employment status and health care funding or eligibility do not belong together. It was started by President Roosevelt in 1942 to attract workers when there was a shortage of employees. Those conditions do not exist in this time of high unemployment. However, I like the fact that it will be a non-profit mutual insurance system, completely separate from the government.

Chapter 26: Reforming the Canadian HealthCare System

The Manitoba Pharmacare Prototype

In 1994, some brainy Manitoba planners conceived the current version of Pharmacare. Applying portions of the successful Pharmacare model to the administration of the other three major healthcare components; that is, the hospital, medical and personal care home systems would improve the Canadian healthcare structure overnight.

Whenever I walk into a Canadian pharmacy, I am struck by the retailer's consumer-service dedication. Pharmacies engage in spirited, free-market competition. Some offer an Advantage card, some "air-miles", others gasoline discounts. Some are open 24-hours every day of the year.

Contrast this sparkle with Canada's drab hospitals and clinics. Hospital corridors are crowded with patients on gurneys, unused equipment strewn everywhere (literally a fire-trap) and men and women housed together in the same hospital room – depressing to see.

The Funding of Medicare

Manitoba residents would have to get used to terms like extra-billing, premiums, and deductibles.

a. Extra-billing

The reason physicians and hospitals extra-bill is because Medicare remittances are inadequate, often just barely enough to stay in business and not enough to make a reasonable profit.

If providers elect to accept the Medicare benefit level as payment in full they could agree to "assignment". This means the Medicare check would be deposited directly into the provider's bank account. If assignment has been agreed to there would be no extra-billing permitted. The advantage for the provider is there are no bad debts and no cost of collecting.

On the other hand, the provider might decline "assignment" and wish to extra-bill. The Medicare check then goes to the patient. Providers of healthcare services would be able to extra-bill if they think the patient can afford to pay more on his own. The decision to accept assignment should be made on a case by case basis.

However, I would like to see a ceiling above which extra-billing is not permitted. For those paying no income tax there should be no extra-billing. But, for example, if the client had $5,000 taxable income last year, extra billing should be allowed up to the point where authorized medical expenses for the year have reached $5,000. After that point, the provider would have to accept the Medicare rate as full payment. For someone with $100,000 taxable income, extra-billing would be allowed up to $100,000, but not after that.

The extra-billing privilege would therefore be limited. Excessive extra-billing could be appealed to the Fee Arbitration Committee of the licensing body, the College of Physicians and Surgeons. Their decision would be binding.

Once the taxable income threshold has been exceeded, a Medicare "Explanation of Benefits" report to the patient would state, "The balance charged by the provider does not need to be paid". This is where there is a stark difference between extra-billing and co-pay. Co-pay has no ceiling and makes no concession for ability to pay.

Financial information from Revenue Canada should only be shared with Medicare. The provider would be oblivious of the client's financial status. There should be no discrimination on the basis of income or two-tier medicine.

Every client would be furnished with an "Explanation of Benefits" by Medicare after every contact with a provider. The public should always be told what has been paid on their behalf. If the extra-billing threshold has been exceeded, the explanation of benefits form would advise the clients that it does not need to be paid.

b. Premiums

As far as premiums are concerned, patients with no taxable income would pay no premium. Their premium would be subsidized 100% by the government.

A premium maximum would be arrived at by an estimate, furnished by qualified actuaries, of what the healthcare insurance would cost in the open market. In Manitoba, in 2014, the cost of healthcare for a family of four was estimated to be $10, 591. This should be set as the full amount of the premium.

The level where the full premium kicks in would be a political decision by the government. It should be a sliding scale from a point where the entire burden is paid by the government to where there is no subsidy at all. The steeper the decline of the slope, the lesser would be the amount necessary to come from general government revenues. A taxable income level of $100,000 might be a good ceiling.

c. Deductible

The great Premier Tommy Douglas from Saskatchewan, the acknowledged founder of Canadian Medicare, always thought there should be a deductible to dissuade clients from wasting precious Medicare resources for frivolous reasons.

The deductible for US Medicare Part B in the US is $147. This sounds about the right amount for someone without any taxable income. This would be enough to dissuade someone from going to a doctor to get a prescription for Tylenol, which is available at lower cost "over the counter".

The maximum level of the deductible and the threshold where it is reached should be a political decision by the government. Perhaps a $5,000 maximum deductible at a taxable income level of $100,000 would be appropriate. There should be a sliding scale between a $147 dollar deductible at the no taxable income level to $5,000 at the taxable income level of $100,000 level (if that were chosen as the target).

With Manitoba Pharmacare the slope of the deductible gets steeper until the $100,000 taxable income level is reached. After that it levels off at 6.36% and continues like that indefinitely. This could result in a deductible so high there would be virtually no coverage for these people. Mind you, they can afford to pay for almost everything on their own. They would still have the benefit of catastrophe coverage if they needed something really expensive, like a heart transplant.

Maybe it should be like Manitoba Pharmacare with no ceiling to the deductible. It would be a political decision.

No Provincial Sales Tax (PST)

In 2014, spending on healthcare in Manitoba was 5.7 Billion dollars. The 8% provincial sales tax (PST) revenue raised around 4 Billion dollars. Most of the PST income is spent on Medicare. The Federal healthcare transfer payment is currently set at 28%, or $1.2 Billion dollars.

Since Medicare would be paid for by premiums the PST could therefore be eliminated, or at least greatly reduced. It might be only one or two percent to cover the subsidy for lower income earners. There is only an additional $500 Million needed to balance the books. How does a PST of only one or two percent sound to the reader?

Fee for Service Billing

All the hospitals and personal care homes would begin to bill on a fee for service basis.

In the US, hospitals bill Medicare and the insurance companies using a bundled account, called the Diagnosis Related Group (DRG) system. There is no need to reinvent the wheel. The DRG system of fee for service Medicare billing has served the American hospital system very well for over 50 years. It should be adopted as the fee schedule for Manitoba hospitals, but with appropriate local charges.

Competition

There would be competition between hospitals. Personal care homes would advertise for clients.

The clients would be treated by the institutions as valued guests and their fee settlement the sole source of revenue. There would be no expectation by providers of receiving any government grants.

Elite Providers

Finally, there should be 'Elite Providers'. These individuals and institutions would not be bound by any Medicare contract. Access to an elite provider would be on the basis of a physician referral and preclearance by Medicare. The total cost of care would be borne by Medicare, no deductible or co-pay.

An institution like The Mayo Clinic in Rochester, MN would qualify as an elite provider.

Patients going to the elite clinic without pre-clearance would only qualify for Medicare coverage. Any additional charges would be on their own dime. Elite providers would require clients to sign an approval form that extraordinary billing has been agreed to.

Government Regulation of Medicare

Clients should be asked to fill out a patient satisfaction form after every encounter with the healthcare service. This would be the cornerstone for government oversight.

A spreadsheet of client feedback, showing a comparison of satisfaction, would be shared with the caregivers. If they were smart, the laggards would shape up. If they were unwilling, or unable to improve their performance, regulation would force them out of business. The patient satisfaction report would concentrate heavily on the professionalism and proficiency of the provider. Did he take time to listen? Was the examination thorough and were the findings discussed in detail? Did the provider offer alternative treatments? If the condition was serious, was there an offer to get a second opinion? All these things are expected from a competent physician. Poor performance by providers should never be tolerated. Those wishing to take short-cuts and "churn" patients or tender inappropriate high billings would be identified and prevented from doing business. The patient satisfaction forms would identify any miscreants.

In addition to the all-important patient satisfaction surveys, there should be an annual on-site inspection of all hospitals, personal care homes and clinics. The physical appearance of the facility must meet minimum standards. Nationally agreed to benchmarks for treatment and ER services must be met. Hallway medicine should be prohibited. Instruments must be properly cared for and not outdated. Just like in every public elevator, there should be a certificate of inspection posted in a public area in every facility. There should also be unannounced visits if there were any complaints from the public.

Family practitioners should have much more freedom to do procedures, especially in rural areas. An attempt should be made to broaden their activities into doing uncomplicated obstetrics, scoping and minor surgery to make their jobs more interesting and to convenience the needs of the public.

I would recommend screening for cancer with all the latest technologies, whether proven to be efficacious or not. The current evidence-based guidelines for cancer screening are repressive and harmful and should be replaced by professional wisdom and good common sense. Doctors are smart enough to interpret the screening data and act on it appropriately.

Nurse practitioners and Physician's Assistants should be doing the work many medical practitioners do today. They would offer diagnostic services, look after minor medical problems, order tests as required and prescribe treatments and prescriptions. They could practice solo, but more frequently work in association with physicians. Their charges would be based on the physician's fee schedule, pro-rated at approximately 85%. Their performance would be subject to government regulation.

Midwives should bill Medicare on a fee- for-service basis. Medicare should compensate midwives at a rate set at 85% of what a physician gets. The presence of midwives should be welcome in the hospitals. If it is a home delivery there has to be a credit equivalent to the cost of a hospital delivery.

Politics

Politics should be removed from the healthcare system. There should be no more favors dispensed as a reward for political support. Examples of political "pork" advanced to a vocal minority would be the "white elephant" known as the Birthing Centre in St. Vital and the unseemly rivalry between hospitals in St. Anne and Steinbach, MB, small cities located only 15 km apart. There is no objection to having two hospitals close together or a birthing center as long as there is no expectation of any preferential government support.

Finally, rigorous government oversight and regulation is extremely important and needs to be augmented. The government should be there to maintain high standards. This only works if the provider and the regulator are not joined at the hip.

Doctors on Salary

There are many who believe a fee-for-service method of remuneration for physicians, hospitals and personal care homes is outdated. They claim it leads to over servicing and over emphasis on procedures. They maintain a system of salaries might stimulate quality of service over quantity.

Happily, in a free country, if a clinic or hospital think they can make a go of it without incentives, we should not deter them. American HMOs have found this doesn't work. But they shouldn't expect patrons of free-enterprise clinics to pay for their mistakes and losses.

Patients should never find themselves locked into a provider network, as patient/doctor relationships do not always remain congenial. Patients should always be able to get a second opinion or switch doctors.

Shopping for HealthCare

How do you go about shopping for a gallbladder operation? The same way you shop for anything else. You ask how much he charges, the same as you do when you go for oil change on your car. If he extra-bills you consider credentials and experience and where he has hospital privileges. It might be worth it to pay extra.

You can also consult the Consumers Reports', *Health Care Blue Book* and compare the quoted fees with the average amount insurance companies pay in your community. This can be a powerful bargaining device.

Lastly, if you Google the doctor's name on the internet there are numerous postings documenting feed-back from previous patients.

Single-Tier System

A single-tier system of healthcare access and quality is the idea that charms advocates of socialized medicine more than anything else. Canada carries this concept to the utmost extreme. So much so, they make it illegal to purchase healthcare with your own money in an open free market. Providers of fee-for-service healthcare outside the healthcare system are subject to be closed by the government.

Unfortunately, despite all that, Canadians with better connections usually jump the queue. Members of parliament in Ottawa, and workers under the compensation board or disability insurance all skip past the queue. The single-tier concept has conspicuous bumps and pit-falls.

A much better way of getting a single tier system would be if there was a strong free-market economy and the queue did not exist. If there were no wait lists and no barriers to access, you would have the perfect single- tier system. American consumers of healthcare get a blank look in their eyes when a two-tier healthcare system is mentioned. There are no wait lists except in the VA system.

Physician Administrators

Canadian hospitals will not allow actively practicing physicians to sit on hospital boards because they are presumed to have a vested interest. That is a real shame. Doctors are closer to the patients than anyone else. Their input in policy should be considered invaluable.

Physicians are hired by patients to be their advocates. What good is it if the primary patient promoter is kept out of the chamber? Enlightened healthcare institutions in the US insist on having practicing doctors on the board. More than half of the board of the Mayo Clinic is practicing doctors. The head of the board is always a doctor and has to practice at least 25% of the time.

Paying for Privatization

There is a widespread assumption privatization of the healthcare system would cost more. I don't believe that for a minute. The free-market always reduces cost. Early diagnosis and timely treatment with the object of cure has merit for economic reasons, quite apart from the moral grounds. Late treatment is more extensive and expensive. In cancer cases there may be a need to augment surgery with radiotherapy, chemotherapy, and the cost of dying.

Private Clinics

The transition to a national social healthcare insurance system in Canada could take years. Private enterprise should not be squelched in the short-term. The current load on the government-managed healthcare system needs to be lightened.

Dr. Brian Day of Vancouver, British Columbia (former president of the Canadian Medical Association), is experimenting with an entrepreneurial healthcare clinics. Clinics like his are inviting the government to react with a court challenge.

As of August 2012, an injunction has been issued ordering Dr. Day to close his British Columbia private clinic.* The case will likely proceed all the way to the Supreme Court of Canada. Hopefully, the courts will find the ban on private healthcare (use of personal money for medical purposes) in Canada unconstitutional, in keeping with the Canadian Charter of Rights and Freedoms.

Vociferous opponents to this growing private healthcare development are screaming "foul". They view the expansion of Dr. Day's clinic as the thin edge of the wedge, threatening to destroy Canada's single-tier universal healthcare system. Moreover, they claim the private system may take the best doctors from the public system. Therefore the public system could have even longer wait lists and inferior services.

These private clinics are currently designed to meet the needs of government agencies like the Workers Compensation Board and private insurance companies that provide disability insurance. When there

---

*   *Canadian Press, August 23, 2012.*

is a workplace injury or disability claim the insurer presses for medical testing as soon as possible. Claimants are on disability leave and compensation until the claim is resolved.

Hence, employees with work-related minor elective complaints can be triaged ahead of a patient suspected of having cancer. This does not sound like single-tier medicine to me.

In Manitoba, a private healthcare facility (The Pan-Am Clinic) was snuffed out as a private entity in 2001, not through the courts, but via the government buying the facility.* It now operates as a government-managed facility.

In the province of Quebec a court challenge to the government healthcare monopoly proved successful (*The Council of Canadians*, May 19, 2011).** Referring to the Quebec Charter of Rights and Freedoms, the Supreme Court of Quebec ruled the Quebec government has no right to forbid Quebeckers from using their own money to purchase healthcare from accredited provincial providers.

It is still illegal to operate a private healthcare facility in the rest of Canada.

Second-Tier Emerging

The Mayo Clinic (headquartered in Rochester, Minnesota) is striving to capitalize on the Canadian desire for more expeditious healthcare services. With a new office in Calgary, Alberta, Mayo now markets its own brand of healthcare to Canadians. Also, the Mayo Clinic is cementing an association with the Altru Clinic in Grand Forks, North Dakota, offering convenient services to residents of Manitoba, Saskatchewan and Northwestern Ontario. American

---

*   *Eroding Public Medicare Oct. 6, 2008.*
** *Council of Canadians. May 19, 2011*

private institutions are creating the second-tier of healthcare, whether Canadians like it or not.

Australia ushered in a two-tier medical care system that now appears to be starving the public system.* Those that can pay are apparently being forced into the private system. A Pharmacare type of insurance system would keep the people with no taxable income from being disadvantaged.

A Manitoba study showed ophthalmologists with public system privileges, who also own private facilities, are pressuring patients into private care.** This misrepresents the motives of the ophthalmologists. A two year waiting list for an intraocular lens is a long time. If the patient wants to purchase the lens himself and get it done next week seems like a logical decision the patient should be allowed to make. What's wrong with freedom of choice?

Taiwanese Healthcare System

Taiwan adopted the Canadian idea of a single-payer government universal healthcare insurance system but without the government-managed component. The plan resembles standard Medicare in the United States except it applies to all age groups in the country, covering virtually everyone. All medical conditions are covered, as are pharmaceuticals and even Chinese herbal remedies.

The Taiwanese system offers compelling evidence a free-enterprise universal healthcare system funded by social health insurance is both feasible and offers high quality care. Under the Taiwanese model, providers operate as independent entities; there is no direct government funding or control. There is freedom of choice. There are no

---

*   *Medical Journal of Australia*, vol. 107, 2007.
** *Eroding Public Medicare*, OCT 8, 2008.

wait lists. Providers bill the government and are paid electronically within 24 hours.

According to Uwe E. Reinhart, Professor of Political Economy at Princeton University,* Taiwan spends only 2% of the system's healthcare budget on administration.

About half the hospitals interface electronically with each other, sharing medical records. By 2016, all Taiwan hospitals are slated to be virtually connected. Physicians can access patients' previous medical records, such as hospital discharge summaries and medication history instantly from any other provider in the country. By simply swiping the patient's medical card on his computer, all his/her encoded information is immediately displayed. Time and money are saved as the potential duplication of medical tests is eliminated via instant medical information sharing.

Fierce competition between health care providers is encouraged. Clinics emphasize customer service, offering long hours, supplying complementary transportation for seniors, and so on. Competition keeps costs down. Taiwan's 23,000,000 citizens enjoy what is possibly the best healthcare system in the world.

The beauty about the Taiwanese system is providers consider patients an asset rather than an expense – in sharp contrast to the Canadian healthcare approach. All the difficulties in the Canadian system with long wait lists, hallway medicine, deteriorating infrastructure, surly workforce behavior, waste, and politically motivated funding disparities are eliminated once and for all. It becomes a consumer oriented healthcare system.

However, no system is perfect. Even the near-ideal Taiwanese health care system shows cracks that need to be fixed. Firstly, premiums are partly employer-based (60%) which we know creates

---

*   *NY Times, July 27, 2012.*

problems when there is high unemployment. Secondly, current Taiwan medical premiums are not high enough, causing a healthcare deficit. Thirdly, according to T. R. Reid, evidence shows providers are over-servicing patients, often cutting time spent with patients to five-minute sessions ("churning"), favoring quantity over quality of patient visits. Resources are wasted as a result. More regulation is obviously needed. I would recommend patient satisfaction forms be used. Lastly, it would be preferable if the insurer were a single-payer independent non-profit corporation, not so closely allied with the policing authority. The Taiwanese single-payer universal government healthcare insurance program would therefore benefit from a Manitoba Pharmacare-like variation.

Opposition to Social Health Insurance System

In Canada there would be vigorous objection to a change from socialized medicine to social healthcare insurance. Opposition to privatization would be voluble and brutal.

Labor unions fear privatization. Many medical procedures would move into private surgery centers, unlikely to be unionized. GFT physicians would not be subsidized and have to compete in the open market with private clinics. The WRHA would become a private insurance company and not need nearly as many employees. All these people have something to lose and would object.

Canada actually has one great advantage when it comes to healthcare reform. Since there is virtually no commercial healthcare insurance business anymore, there would be no healthcare industry lobby to contend with. There are no longer many insurance company employees that might be displaced or losing their jobs.

Since the previous healthcare institutions are still intact, there would be no problems with returning assets to the original corporate owners. There is no need to divvy up the possessions of the various healthcare resources on an arbitrary basis.

*T.R. Reid, *The Healing of America*, Penguin, 2009.

Other Attempts at Social Health Insurance

Jeffrey Simpson (*Chronic Condition*, Penguin Group, Canada, 2012) writes, a Pharmacare-style plan has been proposed before - at a Liberal party rally in 1961. Delegates at that meeting proposed a healthcare plan that would provide free access to those below a certain taxable income level. Those above that baseline would pay a deductible, relative to their marginal tax rate. The delegates rejected this proposal due to the possibility the rich would be doubly taxed, first by the deductible and also through general income taxation. They obviously could not cope with the situation that exists today, where the Old Age Pension gets clawed back to the last dollar from seniors with a taxable annual income of $120,000. "Times are changing."

Questions and Answers

I was invited to share my thoughts on reforming the Manitoba healthcare system at a Service Club meeting. I began by describing what the future Canadian healthcare system should look like.

There should be a universal. single-payer, private, non-profit, Mutual, social healthcare insurance system at arm's length from the government to serve everyone from the cradle to the grave. By calling it Mutual, I envisage a company with no shareholders. Any profits would be returned to the clients by rebates or reduced premiums.

Government interaction with the non-profit corporation (let's call it Medicare) should be limited to oversight, regulation and premium subsidy for those with low taxable income - and nothing more.

I described the evolution of Canada's social healthcare insurance system in the fifties to government-managed healthcare in the early 1970s. I described the holiday bed closures, the warehousing of patients, the last minute cancellations, the rationing, the shortage of equipment and manpower, the wait lists, the unnecessary suffering, the disease progression and the avoidable mortality. Afterwards, there was a question and answer session.

The first person wanted to know how you would attract doctors to practice in the inner-city, where there might be fewer people earning enough money to be extra-billed? I replied, "The young doctor working in the underserved inner-city would probably build up a busy practice much quicker. He might be making a good living with a busy practice while his colleague in the suburbs is still struggling to attract clients. Extra-billing would drive some clients away."

Somebody had heard in the US there is a new system of doctor compensation called "Performance Based Compensation". I answered, "In this method of remuneration, physicians are rewarded, or given bonuses, if their patients have better outcomes. For example, there would be a reward if diabetes or heart failure is managed better than average." "The idea behind this is to improve physician performance by tempting them with a bonus."

I stated, "The doctors practicing in the affluent areas of the city would have more compliant patients, better luck with performance-based compensation and get all the bonuses.

That does not seem fair. Results in the US suggest that performance-based compensation is too complicated to administer properly and does not work."

Someone else wanted to know how the fees would be set. He had heard that in some parts of the US providers do not accept Medicare patients anymore because the fees are too low.

I replied, "Eventually, patients may find doctors and hospitals don't accept Medicare and have to go to the ER for care, where they cannot be refused. However, care in the ER is two or three times more expensive. In addition, it is inappropriate care, being piecemeal, not preventive and not consistent care."

"It is the free market that balances supply and demand. When clients start going to the ER in excessive numbers because doctors are so scarce, Medicare has to adjust physician compensation to increase the supply."

"The free enterprise system always finds a balance between supply and demand. If the government does not 'pony up' with a reasonable fee structure, the supply of doctors dries up."

"The problem with government-managed healthcare is that it is politicized. A decision to adjust fees has to be debated in the legislature. A private corporation can make a decision at a board meeting lasting only 10 minutes. It is a simple business decision."

Someone asked, "Surely a universal healthcare insurance system is going to cost more. How are we going to pay for it?"

I asked him, "Why are you assuming it would cost more. I would expect it would cost much less. You see, the original motive for block funding was to limit the cost of Medicare. However, all that happened was rationing, waste and inefficiency."

"Looking at it realistically, if people pay a portion of the cost themselves, with their deductible, that portion would not come out of the public treasury."

"Undue waiting puts people into a position where they need more expensive treatment, such as radiotherapy, chemotherapy and hospice care for cancer. The old adage still rings true, a stitch in time saves nine.

"Also, if a person pays part of the fee out of his own pocket, as with the deductible, there is an inclination to question the need for the test or to shop around for a lower price. In the US, the average price for any procedure can be found in the *Healthcare Blue Book*."

"Competition always brings prices down. An MRI at my personal physician's office in Mesa costs $2,250. I know the charge across the street is only $950. They advertise the price in the local newspaper. It is the same scanner and the standards are likely the same."

The same person added, "Some might delay going to the doctor if they are subject to a deductible." I replied. "That would be a personal decision. It is one thing to make a poor choice on one's own volition and another to have government failure foist an unwelcome delay on you. In a free country there is freedom to make a poor decision."

A middle-aged gentleman in a business suit asked angrily, "Why are you always using anecdotes to savage the Canadian healthcare system. You have scientific training. You should know better than this. Anecdotes are not representative. They can be misleading and tantamount to scandal mongering."

I replied, "I could not agree more. But show me the research that shows that a long wait list or cancellation of treatment does not lead to suffering and preventable mortality. No one is allowed to do this kind of research. The findings could lead to serious legal consequences for the provider. Obviously, it is not in the best interest of the provider to bring devastating information to public view. For example, it was not a scientific study that revealed that there were 40 deaths while on the waiting list at the government-managed Phoenix Veterans Administration Hospital that led to the

Congressional Hearings in 2015. It was the report of whistle blowers at the Phoenix VA Hospital - anecdotal reports. We have to rely on the the only thing that is available to us. We use anecdotes or we leave things as they are."

Another wanted to know if Canadian Medicare would cover visits to providers in other countries.

"It would be a challenge to Canadian providers if they had to compete with the super-efficient American hospitals and doctors. Cross-border barriers to international health care shopping are there to keep people in Canada."

"We would soon find out if it is cheaper to get good healthcare in Canada, wouldn't we?"

"For retirees, there would no longer be a need for "snowbird" healthcare insurance."

"It should be the same as automobile insurance. No one needs to purchase special insurance when they go on a holiday to Yellowstone Park."

"I would make access to foreign clinics and hospitals the cornerstone of my healthcare system reform. Nothing should deter clients from going south, carrying their Canadian benefits with them. The Canadian fee schedule would remain the same on both sides of the border."

"That would solve the waiting period and hallway medicine problem overnight. If the Canadian clinic cannot do the test for three months you could go to the States and get it done the next day with the full support and blessing of Canadian Medicare. The same would be true for hospitals and personal care homes."

The Single Payer Healthcare System - Faults and Fixes

"Nothing I have said here so far today is more controversial and yet more important. I am advocating an instant solution to all our problems with wait lists and standards of care, in one fell swoop."

Some shook their heads in disagreement. "Listen," I remonstrated with my opponents, "you cannot insist healthcare in Canada is cheaper, or argue it is better, if you have to use coercion to keep patients from going south."

The Chairman got up to close the meeting. However, I asked if I could wind things up with one more observation.

I said, "Don't hold your breath. None of this is going to happen soon without an enormous political struggle."

"The biggest obstacle to reforming the Manitoba Medicare system would be the federal government. They pay 28% of our health care bills through transfer payments, to the tune of 1.23 billion dollars a year in Manitoba. They might decide to withhold their remittances."

"The Federal government has five principles that must be complied with to get cost-sharing. The first condition is the requirement to have a centralized government authority to micro-manage the healthcare system. To get funding you must have socialized medicine! What I am recommending is universal social health insurance. It might not qualify. The other four are not contentious and would be complied with enthusiastically. These are comprehensiveness, portability, accessibility and universality."

The meeting was declared closed. Some hung around to debate the need for a deductible. "Admittedly, this is a touchy subject for most Canadians." I added, "Look, nobody is going to go bankrupt with a small deductible."

It was time to go home.

*Jeffrey Simpson, Chronic Condition, Penguin Group, Canada, 2012.

Conclusion

In Canada, government-managed healthcare (socialized medicine) has led to waste, inefficient care, delayed diagnosis and treatment. As a result the toll in human suffering is incalculable and many hundreds of avoidable deaths are likely each year.

A single-payer universal social health insurance plan similar to American Medicare is my prescription for a happy and healthy Canada and the United States of American.

But, unlike American Medicare, it should be an independent not-for-profit Mutual insurance Corporation corporation subject to government inspection and regulation.

It should provide social insurance coverage from the cradle to the grave.

Curriculum Vitae

Licentiate Medical Council of Canada

Diploma, National Board of Medical Examiners, U.S.A. Fellow Royal College of Surgeons (C)

Certified American Board of Urology

Distinctive Awards:

The winner first Prize Essay, New York Section, American Urology Association, "The Effect of Pudendal Nerve Anesthesia on Urinary Incontinence after Prostatectomy" - April 1964.

Nominated for the Manitoba Order of the Buffalo Hunt.

List of Publications and Presentations

Ferguson, M.F., Krahn H.P., Hildes, J. "Parotid Secretion of Protein in Man" - Canadian Journal of Biochemistry and Physiology 36: 1001, 1958.

Krahn, H.P., Tessler, A.N., and Hotchkiss, R.S. "Studies of the Effect of Hydrocele Upon Scrotal Temperature, Pressure, and Testicular Morphology" - J. of Fertility and Sterility 14: 226, 1963.

Krahn, H.P., Morales, P., Hotchkiss, R.S. "Experience with Tubeless Cystostomy" - Journal of Urology 91: 246 1964.

Krahn, H. P., Morales, P. "The Effect of Pudendal Nerve Anesthesia on Urinary Incontinence after Prostatectomy" -Journal of Urology 94: 282, 1965.

Krahn, H. P., Morales, P., Hotchkiss, R. S. "A Comparison of Suprapubic Prostatectomy With and Without Vesical Neck Closure" -Journal of Urology 96: 83, 1966.

Tessler, A.N., Krahn, H. P. "Varicocele and Testicular Temperature" -Journal of Fertility and Sterility 17: 201, 1966.

Krahn, H. P. "Vesico-ureteral Reflux – Late Results" -Presented Canadian Urology Association Annual Meeting, May, 1967.

Moharib, N.H., Krahn, H. P. "Acute Scrotum in Children with Emphasis on Torsion of Spermatic Cord" -Journal of Urology, 104: 601, 1970.

Krahn, H. P., Axenrod, H. "The Management of Severe Renal Lacerations" -Journal of Urology, 109: 11, 1973.

Krahn, H. P., MacLeod, I. D., Caplan, B., Decter, A. "Complications of Ileal Conduits" - Presented Canadian Urological Association Annual Meeting, June 1972.

San Vicente, P., Krahn, H. P. "The Late Complications of Genitourinary Tract Trauma" Presented Canadian Urological Association Annual Meeting, June 1972.

Bochinsky, B., and Krahn, H. P. "The pitfalls of Renal Angiography in Differential of Renal Masses" Presented Canadian Urological Association Annual Meeting, Vancouver, June 1973.

Lim, A., Caplan, B., Krahn, H. P. "Cystectomy for Bladder Cancer" - Presented Canadian Urological Association Annual Meeting, June 1973.

Mathur, V., Krahn, H. P., Ramsey, E. W. "Total Cystectomy for Bladder Cancer", - Journal of Urology, June, 1981.

Krahn, H. P. "Experience with Tanagho Procedures" -Presented Canadian Urological Association Annual Meeting, June 1987.

Krahn, H. P. "Conservative Treatment of Vesico-vaginal Fistula" -Presented Canadian Urological Association Meeting, June 1987.

Krahn, H. P. "Comparison of Digital Directed and Ultrasound Guided Biopsy of the Prostate Using the Biopty Gun" -Presented Canadian Urological Association Meeting, June 1990.

Krahn, H. P. "The Scope of Ultrasound in General Urology." -Presented American Urological Association Annual Meeting, 1991.

Krahn, H. P. "Transrectal Ultrasound Findings in Prostadynia and Orchalgia." - Presented at the American Urological Association Meeting, 1991.

Krahn, H. P. "Modification of the Mitrofanoff Procedure." -Presented at the Canadian Urological Association Annual Meeting, 1991.

Wong, H., Krahn, H. P. "Concomitant Carcinoma of the Penis and Urethra Treated with a New Method of Continent Diversion" -Journal of Urology, September 1992.

Krahn, H. P. "The Impact of Prostatic Specific Antigen and Transrectal Ultrasound Guided Biopsy (TRUS) in the Diagnosis and Management of Carcinoma of the Prostate", - Presented Canadian Urological Association Annual Meeting, June, 1992.

Krahn, H. P. "Downsizing of Clinical Stage B Carcinoma of the Prostate with Flutamide", -Presented at Science and Medicine Issues and Controversies in Prostate Cancer Meeting, Quebec City, March, 1993.

Krahn, H. P. "Downsizing of Clinical Stage B Carcinoma of the Prostate with Flutamide" -Presented Canadian Urological Association Annual Meeting, June 1993.

Krahn, H. P. "Differential Diagnosis and Medical Management of BPH" -Presented at 39th Annual Meeting of the Royal College of Physicians and Surgeons of Canada, Sept. 1993.

Krahn, H. P. "The Results of Prostatic Specific Antigen Testing (PSA) in Men Age Seventy Years or Less" -Presented at Science and Medicine Canada, Mar. 1994.Krahn,

H. P. The Location of Small Volume Cancer of the Prostate" -Presented at the American Urological Association Annual Meeting 1994.

Krahn, H. P. "The Location of small volume Cancer of the Prostate" -Presented at the Canadian Urological Association Annual Meeting 1994.

Krahn, H. P. "The Results of Finesteride 5 MG/Day (Proscar) for six months for the treatment of Benign Prostatic Hypertrophy (BPH)" -Presented at the Canadian Urological Association Meeting, 1994.

Krahn, H. P. "Downsizing of Clinical Stage B Carcinoma of the Prostate with Flutamide Prior to Radical Prostatectomy" -Presented at Canadian Urological Association Meeting, June, 1994.

Krahn, H. P. "Prostatic Specific Antigen (P.S.A.) Velocity and Gleason Score." Presented at the Canadian Urological Association Annual Meeting, 1994

Krahn, H. P. "The Location of Small Volume Cancer of the Prostate" -Presented at the American Urological Association Annual Meeting in 1994.

Krahn, H. P. "Reresection of Urethra in Cases of Radical Prostatectomy with Positive Margin on Frozen Section" -Presented at Science and Medicine Issues and Controversies, June 1995.

Krahn, H. P., Rifkin, M. N., Crofts, N. G., Kapoor, A. "Pure KTP and combined YAG/KTP Laser Prostatectomy for Benign Prostatic Hypertrophy (BPH)." -Presented at the Canadian Urological Association Annual Meeting, 1995.

Krahn, H. P. "Holmium Laser Assisted Transurethral Resection of the Prostate (TURP)." -Presented at Canadian Urological Association Annual Meeting, June, 1996.

Krahn, H. P. "Transurethral Resection of the Prostate for Benign Prostatic Hyperplasia." -Presented Northeastern Section of American Urological Association, Buffalo, 1996.

Krahn, H. P. "Holmium Laser Assisted Transurethral Resection of the Prostate (TURP) for Benign Prostatic Hyperplasia (BPH)." -Presented at 14th World Congress of Endourology, Melbourne, Australia, Nov. 1996.

Krahn, H. P. Trimedyne Holmium Workshop, Winnipeg, Nov. 1996.

Krahn, H. P. "Progressive Techniques in Holmium Laser Urology Applications Workshop", New Orleans, Louisiana, April, 1997.

Krahn, H. P. "Holmium Laser Transurethral Resection (TURP) for Benign Prostatic Hyperplasia." -American Urology Association Annual Meeting, 1997.

Krahn, H. P. "Is a Routine Transrectal Ultrasound Examination (TRUS) an Essential Part of a Complete Evaluation of the Prostate?" -Presented at the Canadian Urological Association Annual Meeting, 1997.

Krahn, H. P. "Holmium Laser Transurethral Fulguration of Superficial Bladder Tumors" Presented at Canadian Urological Association Annual Meeting, 1997.

Krahn, H. P. "Holmium Laser Transurethral Resection of the Prostate (TURP) for Benign Prostatic Hyperplasia" -Presented Canadian Urological Association Annual Meeting, 1997.

Krahn, H. P. Visiting Professor, Thunder Bay, Ontario, June, 1997.

Krahn, H. P. "Holmium Laser Transurethral Resection of the Prostate (TURP) for Benign Prostatic Hypertrophy (BPH)" -Presented Canadian Urological Association Annual Meeting, June, 1997.

Krahn, H. P. Visiting Professor, Foothills Hospital, Calgary, Alberta, Aug., 1997.

Krahn, H. P. "Holmium Laser Fulguration Multiple Superficial Bladder Tumors" - Presented at 15th World Congress on Endourology, Edinburgh, Scotland, Aug., 1997.

Krahn, H. P. "Holmium Laser Transurethral Resection of the Prostate (TURP) for Benign Prostatic Hyperplasia (BPH) Presented at 15th World Congress on Endourology, Edinburgh, Scotland, Aug. 1997.

Krahn, H. P. "Fulguration of Superficial Bladder Tumors" -Presented at 15th World Congress of Endourology, Edinburgh, Scotland, Aug., 1997.

Krahn, H. P. "Holmium Laser Fulguration of Carcinoma in Situ of the Bladder" - Presented at 15th World Congress of Endourology, Edinburgh, Scotland, Aug. 1997.

Krahn, H. P. Workshop on Holmium Laser Prostatectomy, St. Andrews, Scotland.

Krahn, H. P. Hands-on Laser Course, Sydney, Australia, Sept. 1997.

Krahn, H. P. Visiting Professor., Dept. of Urology, U. of British Columbia, Oct., 1997.

Krahn, H. P. "Holmium Laser Transurethral Resection" -Presented at Northeastern Section of the American Urology Association, Litchfield, Ariz., Oct., 1997.

Krahn, H. P. "Holmium Laser Applications in Endourology." -Presented at the American Urological Association Annual Meeting, Dallas, Texas, 1997.

Krahn, H. P. Holmium Laser workshop, Dallas, Texas, 1997.

Krahn, H. P. "Holmium Laser Transurethral Resection (HoTURP) for Benign Prostatic Hypertrophy (BPH)." -Presented at the American Urological Association Annual Meeting, 1997.

Krahn, H. P. Holmium Laser Workshop, Feb. 1998, Jakarta, Indonesia.

Krahn, H. P. "Holmium Laser Fulguration of Carcinoma in Situ of the Bladder." - Presented at the American Urological Association Annual Meeting, 1998.

Krahn, H. P. "Holmium Laser Fulguration of Multiple Superficial Bladder Tumors." - Presented at the Annual Meeting of the American Urological Association, 1998.

Krahn, H. P. Holmium Laser Workshop, Abu Dhabi, Arab Emirates, March 1998.

Krahn, H. P. Visiting Professor, U. of Miami, Florida, 1998.

Krahn, H. P. Holmium Laser Workshop, San Diego, Calif. May 1998.

Krahn, H. P. "Holmium Laser Transurethral Resection of the Prostate (HoTURP) for Benign Prostatic Hyperplasia" -Presented at Canadian Urological Association Annual Meeting, June, 1998.

Krahn, H. P. "Holmium Laser Fulguration of Multiple Superficial Bladder Tumors" - Presented Canadian Urological Association Annual Meeting, June, 1998, Nova Scotia.

Krahn, H. P. Holmium Laser Workshop, Jakarta, Indonesia, May, 1998

Krahn, H. P. Video. "Holmium Laser Applications in Endourology", Copyright 1998.

Krahn, H. P. "Holmium Laser Fulguration of Multiple Superficial Bladder Tumors." - Presented World Congress of Endourology, Sao Paulo, Brazil, 2000.

Glezerson, G., Krahn, H. P. "Cost Effectiveness of Holmium Laser Enucleation Prostatectomy." Presented Canadian Urological Association Annual Meeting, 2001.

Glezerson, G., Krahn, H. P. "Cost Effectiveness of Holmium Laser Enucleation Prostatectomy" –Presented European Association of Urology Annual Meeting, Berlin, 2001.

Krahn, H. P., Glezerson, G. "Complications of Holmium Laser Enucleation of the Prostate" -Presented Canadian Urological Association Annual Meeting, 2001.

Krahn, H. P., Glezerson, G. Complications of Holmium Laser Enucleation of the Prostate" –Presented European Association of Urology Annual Meeting, 2001.

Krahn, H. P. "Holmium Laser Fulguration of Superficial Bladder Tumors" -Presented at American Urological Association Meeting, April, 2003.

Krahn, H. P. Holmium Laser Workshop, Jakarta, Indonesia, Feb, 2011

Book Published

Damaged Care – A Surgeon Dissects the Vaunted Canadian and US Healthcare Systems. Published by Friesen Press, 2013.

Praise for *Damaged Care*

"... he makes a convincing case that both the Canadian and US systems could benefit from reforms to make them the same: universal health care based on a single government-provided insurance program that leads clients and health-care providers to shop and compete." - Zach Jordain, Mesa, AZ

"He proposes free care for those who can't afford to pay, and a deductible approach for all others ..." - J. McKinnon, Calgary, AB

"...it's an informative and thought-provoking look into the opaque world of Canadian and US health care." - Waterloo Region Record

"...makes a powerful case for the mismanagement of Canadian health care. It's hard not to be shocked by the insider observations present in this timely and thought-provoking book." – Clarion Review

"...it is a breath of fresh air to read your expose on this monstrous, cold and uncaring government run healthcare!" – V. L. Pizzey, Dugald, MB

"...Provides insights into the healthcare systems of the US and Canada like few others can." "If you really want to know how our health care system in the US compares to the Canadian system, you must read this excellent book." - Dale Walters, Phoenix, AZ

"Now I understand why PSA screening is so important" - John Zacharias, Winnipeg, MB

"I am sure glad I don't live in Canada" – Sue Winslow, Mesa, AZ

About the Author

HENRY P. KRAHN, B.Sc. (MED), M.D. F.R.C.S (C) WAS BORN IN Manitoba, graduated from the University of Manitoba, and trained in urology at New York University's Bellevue Medical Center. He practiced for thirty-eight years in Winnipeg and another eight years with the Mayo Health Care System in Minnesota. He is an associate professor of surgery (emeritus) at the University of Manitoba, was head of urology at the St. Boniface General Hospital in Winnipeg for twenty-three years, and chief of surgery at the Concordia Hospital in Winnipeg for over thirty years. He has been active in medical politics for most of his career, and ran as a Progressive Conservative candidate during the 1977 provincial election in Manitoba. He is the author of a previous book on the Canadian healthcare system entitled *Damaged Care*.

He has been retired since 2011 and lives with his wife in Mesa, Arizona.

Printed in Canada